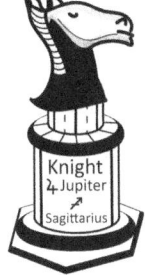

The Planetary Calendar Astrology Companion

Moving Beyond Observation Into Action

Ralph DeAmicis & Lahni DeAmicis

Space and Time Publishing

The Planetary Calendar Astrology Companion
Moving Beyond Observation into Action
By Ralph DeAmicis & Lahni DeAmicis

Published by Planetary Calendar Publishing
An Imprint of Cuore Libre Publishing
Napa, California
www.SpaceAndTime.com
www.PlanetaryCalendar.com

Copyright 2020 Ralph & Lahni De Amicis
ISBN 978-1-931163-68-2
No part of this book may be reproduced in any form without permission from the publisher.

Illustrations: Ralph DeAmicis
Cover Photo; Thanks to
NASA's Photo Galleries, Jet Propulsion Laboratory
and the Big Guy, Jupiter

About the Design: This book was designed to be easy to use. The fonts and spacing are larger than average. The writing style uses shorter sentences, paragraphs and chapters. Fewer words are split between sentences and related ones are generally on the same line. Paragraphs are separated by spaces to make finding your place easier, especially when consulting back and forth with the graphics. Because Astrology is a visual, geometric art with its own alphabet, there are 118 large and detailed graphics and the important ones are repeated, so they'll be where you need them. We have put ergonomics over aesthetics, because Astrology is hard enough to learn without the book design getting in the way. Wishing you enjoyment and illumination in your quest for knowledge. Ralph & Lahni DeAmicis

Contents

Introduction: The Reason for this Book 5

Chapter 1: What is Astrology? Understanding the Three Parts 7

Chapter 2: The Planets as Players 15

Chapter 3: The Signs as Actions 27

Chapter 4: The Whole Sign House System 39

Chapter 5: The Houses as Place 43

Chapter 6: Traditional vs Modern Planetary Rulers 61

Chapter 7: The Table of Dignities 67

Chapter 8: The Aspects, the Transits & You 79

Chapter 9: About Calendars, Seasons & Forecasts 89

Chapter 10: Sun Sign Spaces 95

Chapter 11: The Secret Power in Local Space Charts 107

Chapter 12: Calendrical Healing 115

Chapter 13: Essential Oils as Astrological Tools 121

Chapter 14: The Twelve Terrestrial Houses 131

Chapter 15: The Chinese Elements Explained 141

Chapter 16: The Visible Planets & the Invisible You 149

Chapter 17: The Astrology of Fine Wine 159

Directory of Educational Videos 167

Catalog of Books & Calendars 169

About the Authors 170

Order the Planetary Calendar 172

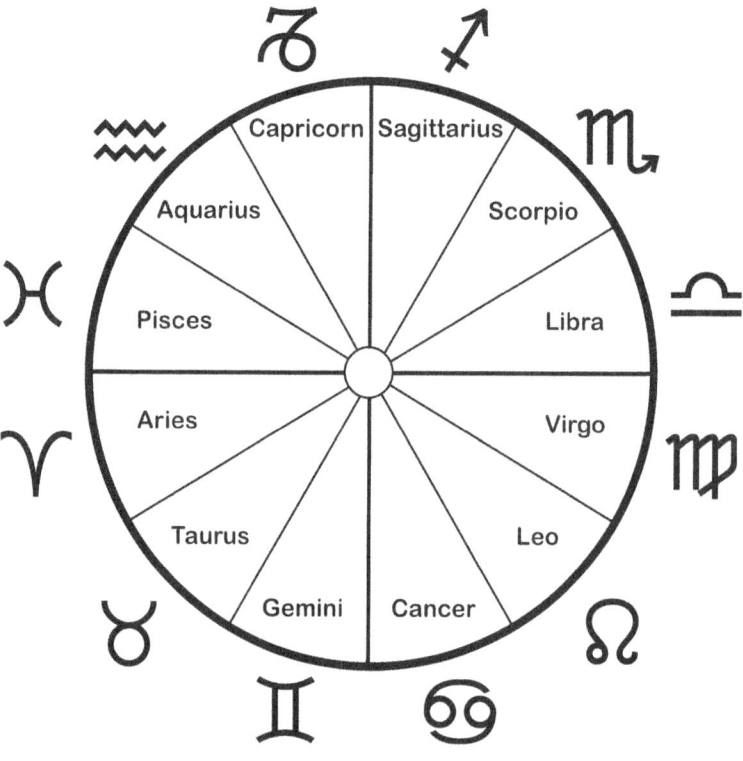

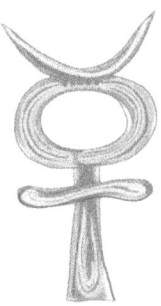

Introduction: The Reason for this Book

This book started as a mini astrology course that was supposed to be built into the new Day Planner that we were designing for our Planetary Calendar. This was a big thing for us. We became the Calendar's authors in 2002, and then its publishers as well in 2017, when we first envisioned a planner. And now for the 2020 edition, for the first time after seventy years of annual publications, the Planetary Calendar would be available in this incredibly handy format, that admittedly, we had to create from scratch.

What could possibly go wrong? After all, we had created numerous books, although we had never designed an Astrological Day Planner before. Let's say we were a tad optimistic about how we were going to fit in these short, to the point chapters.

Then gradually, as the planner got fatter, and fatter, we realized there wasn't room for the mini-course, which itself had expanded to fourteen chapters, including forty plus illustrations. Fortunately designing an astrology book is a lot easier than a planner, so we turned it into its own book, intending it as a kind of companion to the Calendar, someplace between a cousin and a best friend.

We titled it 'Planetary Calendar Astrology' stemming from the fact that it started as a way to help Calendar fans use Astrological transits more effectively in their lives. Doing that requires a grounding in the four basic principles; Planets, Signs, Houses and Aspects, which is exactly how the book starts, introducing these concepts in an illustrative, storytelling style, that we hope you find entertaining.

But that's not enough content for a book, especially when the chapters are short, so the following chapters explore techniques that move you beyond simple observation into strategic action, which is our style of practicing astrology.

As we worked on the book, we realized there were other ways to use these techniques in sync with the Calendar, to help people maintain their vitality and when needed, clear their surroundings and heal their lives.

It resulted in a system that we created for the 2020 Planetary Calendar edition that we call the 'Calendrical Healing System'. It combines Astrology, Meditation, Feng Shui and Herbology, aka plant magic, and it's explained in a three-chapter section. This is one of the places where the book truly serves as the Calendar's companion and when the two are used together, they can yield wonderful insights and benefits every day.

We think the book stands well on its own and it is especially helpful these days when many people are learning Astrology piecemeal online. To turn the art into a lifelong tool, it's necessary to know the foundations and this book provides those in a very friendly manner.

Note: Astrological Terms are Capitalized.

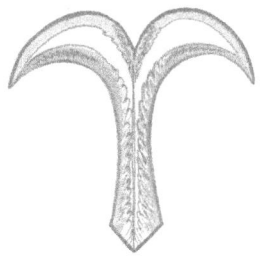

Chapter One: What is Astrology?

Understanding the Three Parts

Note: For the beginner this overview of the Planetary Geometry can be difficult to understand the first time around. So, read it lightly and move onto the 'parts', which are easier to connect with, because they are about 'people'. Then reread this once you feel comfortable with the parts and it will make more sense.

For many centuries Astrology was the pursuit of the most educated, because it requires literacy, mathematics, philosophy and the sciences. It was used for practical, economic, agricultural and political purposes. In some people's minds Astrology is equated with psychics and fortunetellers because it probes that which is not easily seen. But, unlike those talents which depend on accessing the intuition, Astrology is about the symbolic interpretation of observable and predictable phenomena in the heavens and on Earth. It doesn't mean that Astrologers are not intuitive, of course, they're humans. But they depend on the personal Star map to guide them.

The most ancient form of Astrology that we know from archaeological evidence are location-based, and it was used for determining property lines and the orientation of important buildings. Even though Astrology took on a psychological perspective starting in the 20th century, its foundations are geometric and more related to navigation and map making than to psychotherapy.

Astrology is the art of understanding the natural cycles that create our sense of time. Because Planetary cycles are sequential and predictable Astronomers and mathematicians can accurately foretell where the Planets will be in the future. This math is incredibly complicated because we are making our observations from a moving Planet, within the moving Solar System, while the Star we orbit around is itself orbiting around the center of our Galaxy, dragging us along.

This changing perspective produces seemingly non-sequential events, like Planetary Retrogrades, where Planets appear to move backwards in the sky. But even those, like Lunations and Eclipses, and all kinds of configurations are predictable. Using the symbolism of the Planets, and research about historical events during previous similar configurations, Astrologers project scenarios for the future.

Even though humans are amazingly good at plotting the movements of the Planets from our little corner of the Galaxy, Astronomers know there are unknowns at work. Some cosmic intruder, such as a Comet, could disrupt the precise clockwork of our little Solar System. Admittedly, this hasn't occurred in recorded history, although there are stories! In any case it's good to remember that prediction is a dependable, yet imperfect art!

What makes Astrology fun is that the Planets, the most obvious moving parts of this system, are not created equally. Each Planet's cycle is different due to their distance from the Sun and each has a unique influence on the Earth due to their unique chemistry and electromagnetic signatures.

Imagine them as radio and TV stations, each broadcasting their own message, with both daytime and nighttime programming. Venus would be the Home and Garden channel during the day, and then Project Runway at night. Mercury would be the daytime News and then the nightly entertainment gossip shows. Mars would be sports followed by cop shows. Jupiter would be Court TV followed by the Travel Channel. Saturn would be Bloomberg Business News and the Tech Shows. The Moon would be the Soap Operas during the day and the situation comedies at night. The Sun would be the Weather Channel during the day and the Blockbuster movies in the evening.

We watch different shows for different reasons and they don't exist in isolation. The relationships between the Planets are as complex as the dynamics found among families, friends and co-workers. Even though the Planetary motions are predictable, their interaction evolves, always producing unique patterns.

The Chart of the United States of America

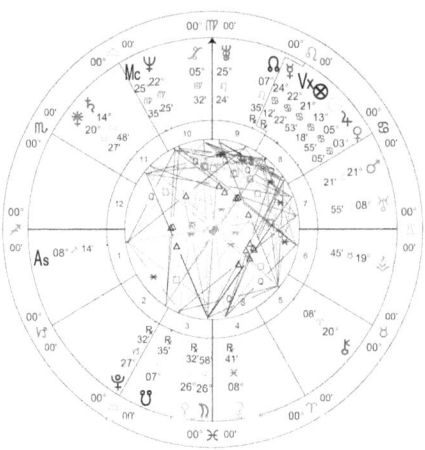

An Astrological Chart captures one fleeting moment, one pattern which will never repeat. Understanding this system requires studying the players and their cycles. Once you understand the personalities that make up the system, you can build on your knowledge as you experience the ongoing movements, or Transits. For example, there is nothing like having Saturn pass over your natal Sun to give you an 'up close and personal' understanding of that Planet. Saturn was always considered the most beautiful of the Angels, but a Transit often makes you feel like you're carrying the weight of the world on your shoulders.

Since ancient times, Astrologers, with the help of craftspeople have been building Astrolabes, mechanical models to describe the motions of the Celestial Bodies. That geometry is a foundational knowledge that one needs to practice Astrology and a three-dimensional model is a great way to comprehend it. But since this book isn't a hologram, we're going to describe that 'clockwork' with words and drawings and hopefully our explanation will add some colorful insights. Before you let the term 'geometry' spook you, don't worry. Today's Astrology computer programs take all the painful math out of the practice. But, if you want to get clues from the moving Cosmos, it helps to understand how it moves.

There are Three Components in an Astrological Chart

The Sun, Moon & Planets

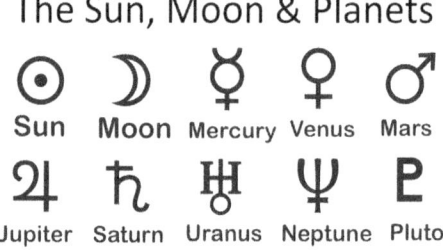

The 12 Signs

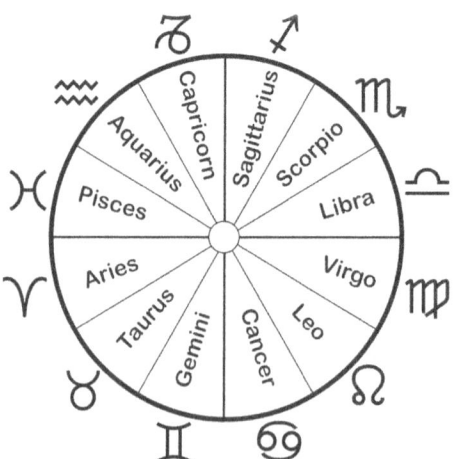

What is Astrology? 11

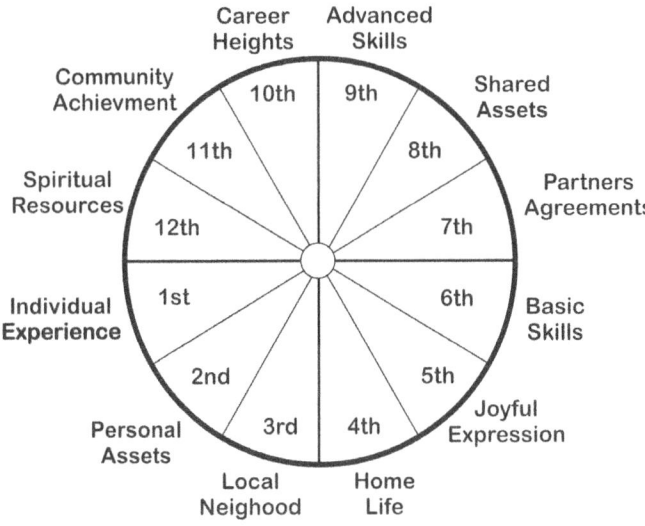

The Ecliptic: The path in the sky along which the appears to Sun travels, accompanied by the Moon and Planets that travel above (north) and below (south) that path. The Ecliptic is tilted at an angle of 23.5 degrees with the Celestial Equator. So, the two intersect at two important places.

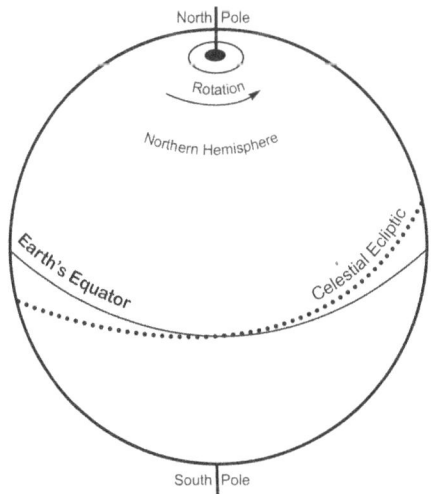

Where the eastern horizon intersects the Ecliptic
The Descendant:
Where the western horizon intersects the Ecliptic

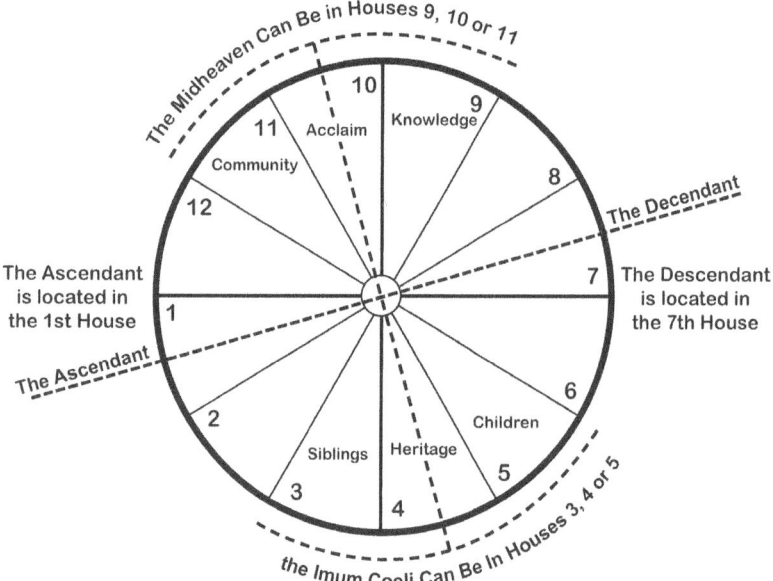

The point of view of the Chart is based on the Houses. They describe where we are standing, the Earth beneath our feet, and they divide the space around us into twelve Houses, using the horizon as their starting reference point. The **Ascendant**, where the Sun rises is to your left. The **Descendant** where the Sun sets is to your right. The spot where the Sun stands at midday along the Ecliptic, called the **Midheaven or MC**, is at the top. The bottom of the Chart is the opposite spot on the Ecliptic, in the sky on the other side of the Earth. So, it is beneath your feet and called the **Imum Coeli, or IC** among friends.

The Signs and Celestial Bodies move in relation to the Houses, and it is comforting to know that in this big spinning clock we call our Solar System, the place where we stand offers at least the illusion of stability.

Western Astrology uses the Tropical Zodiac, which is based on the seasons. That means we divide the circle of the Ecliptic into 360 degrees, or horizontal segments, starting from the spot in the sky where the Sun is on the first day of Spring. That point is called the Vernal Equinox and it describes the position of the Sun traveling along the Ecliptic, as it crosses the Celestial Equator going north. Every day after that the Sun appears to move one more degree.

Clarifying the Confusion

Here is an important point that often causes confusion. Laymen think that we are measuring the motion of the Planets against the twelve Stellar Constellations. But, as we explained above, Western Astrology does not define the location of the Signs according to the Stellar Constellations, that form a backdrop for the Ecliptic, which is called the Sidereal Zodiac. It is used in some advanced Western Astrological techniques, and it is the primary Zodiac in the Vedic Astrology of India.

The West has always used the Tropical Zodiac, probably because of the importance of the seasonal changes for agriculture in northern climates. The Vernal Equinox offers a scientifically verifiable seasonal starting date for the seasons. Because the Sidereal Zodiac gradually changes related to the Vernal Equinox it is used for measuring the Great Ages, but it is at variance with the seasons. Both are valid systems. To put it simply, while the 'Fixed Stars' do play a part in Western Astrology, we are not worrying about that here. End of Clarifying the Confusion.

As we watch the Sun rise each day and move from east to west across the sky, we are also seeing the circle of the twelve Signs rotate overhead, completing a circuit every twenty-four hours. While the Planets change their positions related to the Sign, the Stars are the 'unchanging' backdrop, maintaining their positions in the Signs.

The 360 degrees in that circle are divided into 30 degrees sections that we call the Signs. The Sun moves one degree each day through the twelve Signs, creating the sequence of the seasons and the cycle of growth.

Because the Signs rotate around the location-based Houses, the Chart relates the Cosmos overhead to the moment and spot for which the Chart is 'cast', whether that is for a person (Natal), an organization or an event. If you have ever looked at the heavens and wondered what the Universe is trying to tell you, casting a Chart is a way to find out!

While the Houses and Signs are sequential, with each slice of space and time filling an equal, but progressive role, the Celestial Bodies possess a hierarchy that we see duplicated in our society. This mirroring between the Heavens and our lives on Earth is what the ancient Hermetic saying, "As above so below" describes.

The social structure is crystallized in our mythology and a very accessible model can be found in our Hollywood depicted image of the classic Medieval society, extending from the Royal court; King, Queen, Nobility and Peasants. The next three chapters describe the Planets, Signs and Houses and how they work, starting with the Planets.

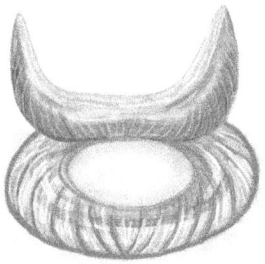

Chapter Two: The Planets as Players

For most of recorded history humans were only aware of the Sun and Moon, called the Lights, and the Planets out to Saturn. The Outer Planets beyond are invisible without a telescope and Astrologers, due to the long orbits of Uranus, Neptune and Pluto, generally consider their influence to be generational. However, we have found them to have specific physiological influences.

For eons, in a world with no electricity to illuminate the long night, the Sun, Moon, Mercury, Venus, Mars, Jupiter and Saturn were the seven players that humans observed crossing the heavens. People used the sky for timing, directions and travel. Escaping slaves heading north followed the handle of the drinking bowl, the Big Dipper, to find Polaris. Hunters and travelers timed their outings with the Full Moon, knowing it would light their path home if they were delayed. Gardeners planted by the Full Moon for the most vigorous sprouts and perfumers harvested at the New Moon to capture the best of those ephemeral oils.

Planetary symbolism abounds in our cultures; in the names for the seven days of the week, Sunday and Monday being the most obvious, and the careful alignment of our historic buildings to gain the favor of the heavens. Most helpfully for our purposes, the Planets are also found in our games and we are going to use the "Game of Kings", Chess, as a wonderful Astrological teaching tool.

The Chess Board

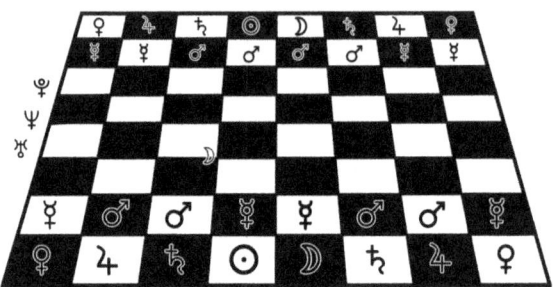

If you have never learned to play chess this is your chance! The pieces on a chess board are based on the Celestial Bodies from the Sun out to Saturn. The sixty-four alternating black and white squares are their battlefield, comprising eight rows of eight squares.

That layout is associated with the 64 Trigrams that describe the year's cycle in the Chinese Book of Changes, the I Ching. The eight spaces relate to the eight compass points in Chinese Astrology and Feng Shui.

While chess reached the West from the Middle East, who found it in India, there are enough echoes of Chinese Astrology in its design to award its creation to the 'Middle Kingdom". Considering that Calcutta was established by the Chinese as a trading port, the connections are pretty obvious.

The goal of chess is to threaten and defeat the **King**, which is called check and checkmate. So, let's start with the King, who represents the **Sun**, that moves one degree a day, mirroring the King who moves one space at a time, in any direction. Because the Planets rotate around the Sun, the King has limited mobility, traveling through the heavens.

In comparison, the **Moon** is the **Queen**. No one rotates around the Moon. Instead the Moon quickly rotates around the Earth, traveling a degree every two and a half hours. This is like a mother whose life revolves around her family. The Queen's speed reflects the Moon's high level of mobility and the Queen can move in any direction, as far across the board as is open, in a single move.

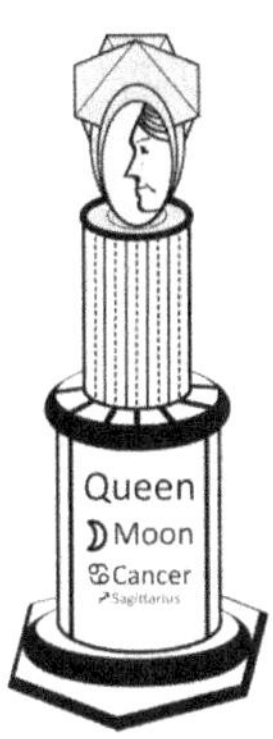

The Queen is the most capable and dangerous piece in the game. If chess is about defending the King, it is equally about using the Queen effectively to accomplish your goals. This mission is symbolic of life where the Sun is your essential spirit, your authentic self which must be defended, by the Moon, your emotional mobility that supplies the capability and motivation necessary to accomplish anything significant. In chess, that means defending the King while vanquishing your opponent. The Moon relates to the Water Sign Cancer and the Fourth House, while the Sun relates to the Fire Sign Leo and the Fifth House.

The Table of Rulers from Chapter Seven

The Table of Rulers Based on the Planetary Triangles

Celestial Body	Dynamic Ruler	Receptive Ruler	Exalted Sign	Dynamic Detriment	Receptive Detriment	Fall Sign
☉	♌	♋ v	♈	♒	♑ v	♎
☾	♐ v	♋	♉	♊ v	♑	♏
☿	♊	♍	♒	♐	♓	♌
♀	♎	♉	♓	♈	♏	♍
♂	♈	♏	♑	♎	♉	♋
♃	♐	♓	♋	♊	♍	♑
♄	♑	♒	♎	♋	♌	♈
⚳	♊	♍	♏	♐	♓	♉

Dotted Line Designates a Primary Sign & V a Vice Sign. www.SpaceAndTime.com (C) 2018 R & L De Amicis

The King and the Queen in chess, like the Sun and the Moon in the Chart, are different from the other players. There is only one King and one Queen, but there are two of each of the other royal pieces, the Bishops (Saturn), the Knights (Jupiter), and the Castles (Venus). There are also the eight Pawns (Mercury and Mars).

This doubling of these three Royals, and the numerous Pawns describes their connection to the Signs, in a system called The Table of Dignities or Rulerships. Being the Ruling Signs means that they are the Celestial Body's most authentic Extroverted expression.

Castle - Knight - Bishop - King - Queen - Bishop - Knight - Castle

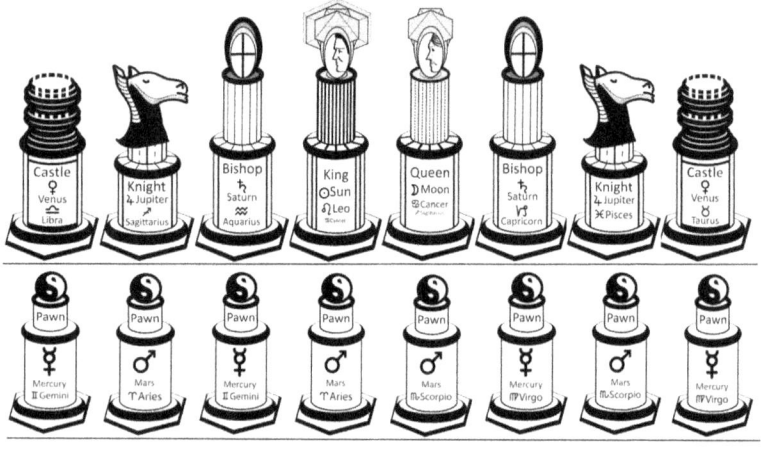

The Eight Mercurial and Martial Pawns

In that system the Lights each rule one Sign. The Sun rules Dynamic Leo (traditionally called masculine) and the Moon rules Receptive Cancer (traditionally called feminine), so they are each other's polarity. But each Planet 'Rules' two Signs; one Dynamic and one Receptive. The Pawns, positioned along the front row, represent the 'common folk' or 'youngsters' of the Planets; Mercury and Mars.

They guard the Royals positioned along the back row. On the board the King and Queen sit at the center of the lineup, each with their own complement of Royals and Pawns to their sides and before them.

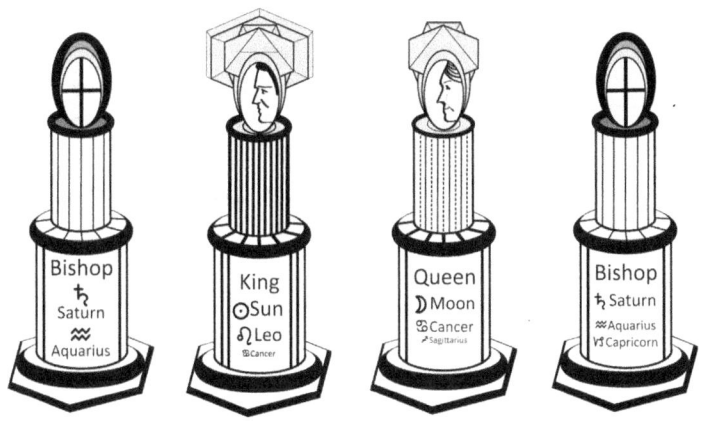

Saturn, Bishops, Aquarius and Capricorn

Beside the King and Queen are the Bishops, representing Saturn. Whenever Royalty is shown sitting on their throne for a formal ceremony, the high priest or priestess is standing by their side to infuse the ritual with the sacred. As one would expect from a priest or priestess, Saturn is a conservative, restrictive, ambitious, serious Planet often connected to time and aging.

It takes twenty-eight years for Saturn to travel through the twelve Signs, spending about two and a half years in each. That was once the average human lifespan. Saturn rules Aquarius (Dynamic) and Capricorn (Receptive), which sit next to each other in the first two months of Winter. This says a lot about the frosty nature of the Planet.

Saturn restricts, so when it returns to the Sign in which a person was born, after twenty-eight years, that is the infamous Saturn Return. It denotes two and a half hard-working, often difficult years that designate the transition from childhood's joys, to adulthood's responsibilities. This compressive cycle repeats every twenty-eight years and it always feels serious. The Earth Sign Capricorn relates to the Tenth House and Air Sign Aquarius relates to the Eleventh House.

Jupiter, Knights, Sagittarius and Pisces

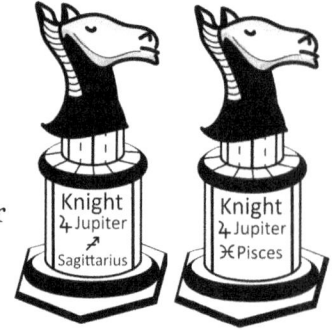

Jupiter expands which describes the entrepreneurial Knights. In chess, the Knight can leap over the other pieces, greatly expanding its capabilities. Jupiter is the largest Planet and tremendously influential as the bringer of luck, travel, education and healing.

The Knight moves at right angles, first two spaces in one direction and then turning right or left for one more space. That 90-degree right angle describes the relationship of the two Signs that Jupiter traditionally rules; Sagittarius (Dynamic) and Pisces (Receptive), which are Square (90 degrees) to each other. This movement describes that angle, or Aspect in Astrology.

Sagittarius and Pisces are the last Signs, respectively, of Fall and Winter so they are both about how humans use the seasonal changes for their personal benefit, while preparing for what is coming. Sagittarius, the Archer Centaur and hunter, takes advantage of the leaves falling, revealing the animals, which are carrying the weight they put on over the warm growing seasons of Summer and Fall. This larder will help carry the family through the Winter season. Pisces uses the coming warmth of Spring to watch for the patches of green amid the melting snow where the sweetest sprouts will be found.

By the Way... Jupiter takes an average of one year to travel through a Sign and twelve years to traverse all twelve Signs, so it expands on the twelve months that make up a year. The twelve

Signs of the Chinese Zodiac are based on the position of Jupiter, although Chinese Astrology's deeper 'Element' system comes from the interrelationship of the cycles of Jupiter and Saturn, the two largest Planets. The Fire Sign Sagittarius relates to the Ninth House and the Water Sign Pisces to the Twelfth House.

Venus, Castle, Taurus and Libra

Next to the Knights, in the corner of the board, are the royal Castles, which represent Venus. They are the secure repository of the wealth, food and other comforts that prosperity provides. That describes the Receptive side of Venus, in the Sign Taurus, which relates to the bounty of the earth, personal talents and attractiveness.

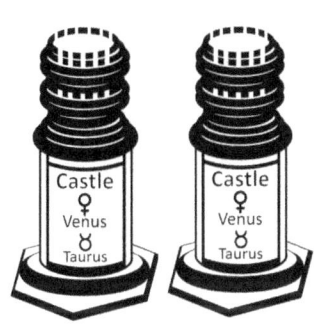

The Castle is also where the courts, records and contracts are kept and that describes the Dynamic side of Venus, the Sign Libra, which rules formal relationships, partnerships and marriages.

The two Signs are separated by a 150-degree Aspect (angle), or what is called a Quincunx, which is considered a trans-dimensional relationship. It bestows the ability to come to conclusions and take actions based on seemingly unrelated information, which is seen as a feminine quality, but is more accurately a Venusian, artistic quality.

This explains why Venus is related to love, which is also a trans-dimensional experience. It transports us between realms. Taurus is the second Sign of Spring and Libra is the First Sign of Fall. Earth Sign Taurus relates to the Second House and Air Sign Libra to the Seventh.

The Pawns Mars & Mercury
Aries and Scorpio - Gemini and Virgo

That brings us to the eight Pawns. They represent the infantry, out there on the front lines. They are the little people that the generals move around the board, and if necessary, sacrifice to attain their greater goal. They relate to the two smallest Planets (other than Pluto), Mercury and Mars, because both have a reputation for boldness and foolishness, venturing into unknown territory with the naivete of youth.

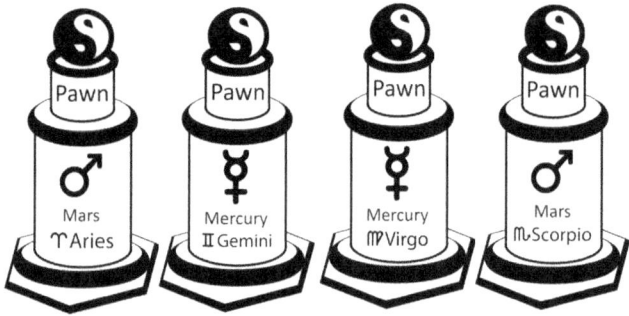

Even though they are similar, Mercury and Mars fulfill very different positions in the Chart. Mercury is the closest Planet to the Sun and is within the orbit of Earth. That means it is always near the Sun King, with a maximum distance of 28 degrees, appearing in either the same Sign as the Sun, or the Sign immediately before or after. Venus also orbits between the Earth and Sun. but can appear as far as two Signs away from the Royal disc.

This solar proximity makes the tiny, reflective Mercury sparkling bright, although it also makes it invisible most of time, with brief appearances periodically near sunrise or sunset.

So, Mercury's relationship with the other Planets is always colored by its dependence, like a secretary, a servant or jester, serving in the shadow of their boss. It also has a close relationship to Venus since they occupy the same environs.

Mars, in comparison, orbits beyond the Earth, so it can appear in any Sign relative to the Sun. It is both more independent and visible, shining like an unmistakable red jewel for longer periods of time, with its brightness varying based on distance and phase. While Mercury is seen as switching his alliance from Sun to Moon with the passing of day and night, Mars is a follower of the Moon, the devoted child of a caring mother. That's because the Moon and Mars come together, in what is called a Conjunction every month, which is how long it takes Luna to traverse all twelve Signs. In comparison, the Sun and Mars are normally Conjunct for only a short time, once a year.

As the smallest Planets, their roles as the Pawns on the chess board make sense. Both Planets are youthful and simpler in their actions than the Royal Planets along the back row. Mercury rules the Signs of Dynamic Gemini and Receptive Virgo, and is the communicator, the nervous system, the collector and dispenser, but not the creator of information. Mars rules Dynamic Aries and Receptive Scorpio and is the aggressor, the actor, the fighter, the hormonal system and the fight or flight response. Both Planets relate to the body's automatic responses, which is why they are the first to encounter new situations. They react quickly and without considering the risk.

The Pawns are on the frontlines, so their actions are simple and limited. Their first move forward can be one of two spaces, then they move one space at a time. They cannot retreat and they can only attack in a forward diagonal. Being hemmed in by such choices, they quickly run out of possible moves, which reflects the limitations of mind and muscle; they will only take you so far.

While their actions are simple and predictable, they are also effective, so other players regularly fall prey to the Pawns. But, just as often, a player sacrifices a Pawn for a greater strategy. The Air Sign Gemini relates to the Third House and the Earth Sign Virgo relates to the Sixth House.

Chess depicts a traditional fortified city. In our historical knowledge of the Planets, Saturn represented the outer walls of that Kingdom, relating to stone and the patience required to build large structures from durable materials. But since 1781 when Uranus was discovered, humanity has become more aware of the powerful players outside of those walls; the outlaws. How do the Planets beyond Saturn fit into this symbolic cosmology? Quite well, especially if we consider what is found outside of the walls of the city, where the streetlights end. The first Planet beyond Saturn is Uranus, which relates to revolutionaries, iconoclasts, innovators and inventors. It is those people and groups that rebel against the traditional ways of doing things.

The discovery of Uranus heralded the huge expansion of technology that moved the world from an agricultural economy to an information society, based on the many manifestations of electricity and physics. Think about Benjamin Franklin, America's most famous Astrologer, flying his kite and key in a lightning storm. That is 'Uranus' at work taking place in the 'New World', flown by a man with no royal heritage or familial financial advantage. Uranus is about every person, the importance of the collective voice, the community. It is no surprise that Astrologers ascribed Uranus to Aquarius because that is the Sign of community efforts.

The thinking of the Astrologers of that era, in assigning Aquarius to Uranus and Pisces to Neptune may have been due to those being the eleventh and twelfth Signs, and thus a higher frequency, so they should relate to the Planets 'beyond' the visible. Pisces, the twelfth Sign, which was associated with the Christian epoch and dissolving the ego, provides a spiritual theme that seems to work for Neptune, the invisible giant beyond Uranus.

Coincidentally, Neptune's discovery in 1846 heralded many important spiritual movements, and social welfare reforms. Hence Neptune has a strong connection to spiritual movements, imagination, visionaries, and compassion for the masses. Spiritual retreats and communities are normally found in remote places, mountains and deserts, far beyond the walls of the towns. Neptune often shows up prominently in the Charts of very successful people because of the importance of having a vision of what you want to accomplish. That imagination is essential to your ability to inspire others to action through your story

Even though astronomers demoted Pluto to a Proto-Planet, Pluto still figures prominently in Astrology Charts. It turns out, after the fact, that the Planet is larger than they originally thought, just a little smaller than Mercury and surrounded by numerous Moons. Pluto's influence may be inhibited by its great distance from Earth, but, on the other hand, Stars, which exist at a much greater distance, are often powerful influences in natal and event Charts. Since there is nothing between Pluto and us but space, maybe its influence is larger than we think. Just ask someone who is having a Pluto Transit over their Sun, Moon or Ascendant.

To depict Pluto in this story, the image of the hermit would work, except that Pluto is not alone, but accompanied by those tiny Moons. So maybe it is the Master of a special skill, like martial arts, surrounded by students. There is a strong sense of obsessive perception with whatever Pluto is focused on and an interest in global issues and long timelines. There is also a sexual component in the Pluto myth, as well as a desire for power and the talent of invisibility. Pluto seems to imbue people with the ability to focus deeply and perceive hidden power and vulnerabilities. A team of deeply committed Ninja makes a wonderful image for this distant Planet and its Moons.

There are other Bodies that influence the interpretations of the Chart. Most prominent are the largest Bodies in the Asteroid Belt that orbit between Mars and Jupiter. The largest is Ceres, which is planet shaped and one fifth the size of Mercury. Three other major asteroids; Vesta, Juno and Pallas Athena appear frequently in Charts and possess well defined meanings.

Beyond the orbit of Saturn is Chiron, a dwarf Planet that probably started its life as a Comet. There is a great deal written about the many asteroids and Fixed Stars used in Astrology. Discovering their influence is one of the joys that keeps studying the art a lifetime pursuit. Next, let's discuss the Signs that color their actions as they travel through our lives.

The Twelve Signs

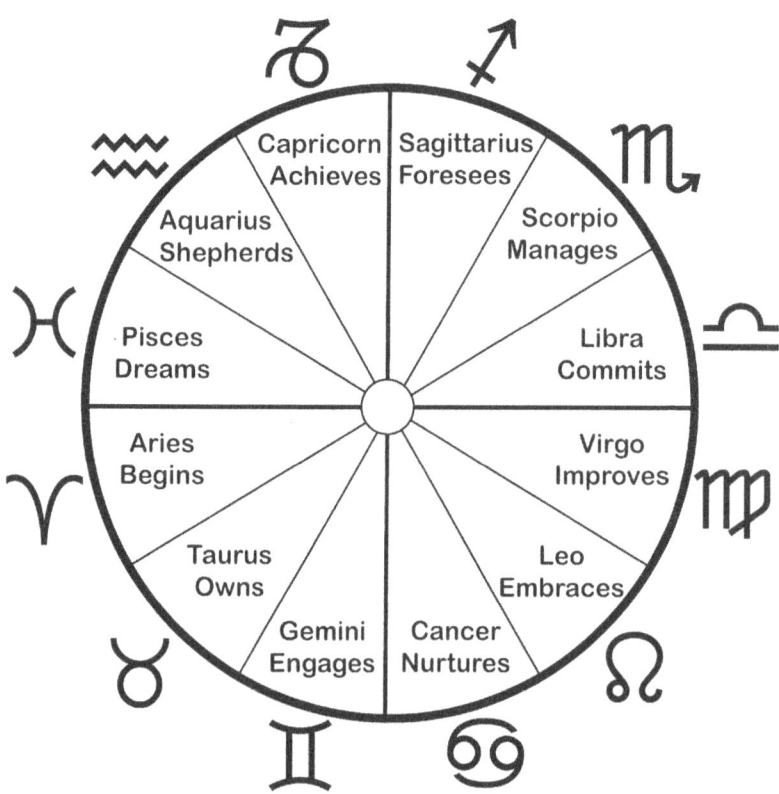

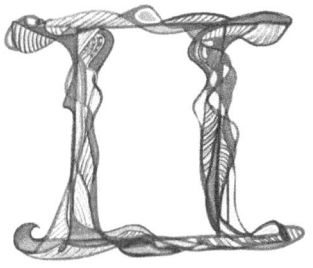

Chapter Three: The Signs as Actions

Almost everyone knows their Sun Sign, or where the Sun was in their chart when they were born. But, do they understand that the twelve Signs describe thirty-degree sections of the path in the sky, called the Ecliptic, where the Sun appears to travel, one degree each day, creating the year?

Because the Ecliptic and Equator are not parallel, but cross at a 23-degree angle, the Sun splits it time between the northern and southern hemispheres, creating the seasons.

The first day of each season is a turning point in the Sun's yearly passage, which most importantly, we experience through the changing length of the day. On the first days of Spring (Vernal Equinox, 1st degree Aries) and Fall (Autumnal Equinox, 1st degree Libra), when the Sun crosses the Equator, the day and night are equal length.

After the Vernal Equinox (Equal Night) each day is longer, until the first day of Summer (Summer Solstice, 1st degree of Cancer). After the Autumnal Equinox each day is shorter, until the first day of Winter (Winter Solstice, 1st Capricorn). What all this means is that the Signs represent time, location and the angle with which the Earth is receiving the Sun's light!

Understanding the Connections Between the Signs

Each season is a quarter segment of that Ecliptic pathway, and each segment is divided into three sections, which are the Signs. The shifting angle of the light in the Sun's apparent annual journey, and its effects on weather, determine the actions that take place during each period. Each thirty-degree Sign builds upon what happened before. For example, during the last third of Winter, Pisces, the thaw makes dissolved nutrients available to the sprouting plants, encouraged to the surface by the warming of Spring, in Aries.

The twelve Signs are equal components in that cycle, related to each other by four criteria that are unique to time and Astrology; Season, Polarity, Element and Quality. This is a little like the four familial connections that humans make to their parents, siblings, mates and children.

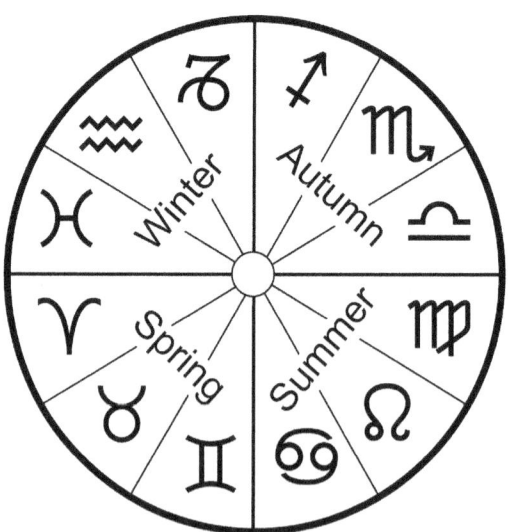

First, What is the Sign's Season: Are they part of Spring, Summer, Fall or Winter? Spring is the season of hope, Summer is the season of fulfillment, Fall is the season of consolidation and Winter is the season of contraction.

The Polarities

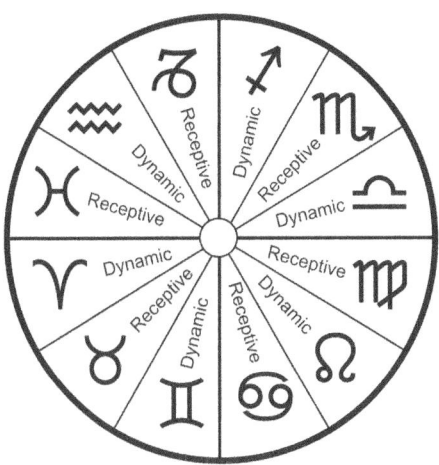

Second, What is The Sign's Polarity? Traditionally the Signs are considered masculine or feminine, alternately, Yang or Yin. But we prefer Dynamic or Receptive, because that describes their action rather than their nature. The Signs start with Dynamic Aries, then Receptive Taurus, Dynamic Gemini, Receptive Cancer, Dynamic Leo, Receptive Virgo, Dynamic Libra, Receptive Scorpio, Dynamic Sagittarius, Receptive Capricorn, Dynamic Aquarius, Receptive Pisces. This tells you whether the energy is Dynamically pushing into the social world or Receptively pulling into the personal world.

Third, What is The Sign's Element? Many people know the four traditional elements that come to us through the ancient Greeks, Fire, Earth, Air and Water. This is not equivalent to our modern Elemental Table, denoting Oxygen, Hydrogen, Zinc, etc. Those ancient elements describe what modern science calls the four states of Matter: Fire equals Plasma, Earth equals Solid, Air equals Gas and Water equals Liquid. The Element describes the Sign's essential 'being' and the way they act in the world. Each Sign within an Element shares that essential nature although they will express it differently depending on their season.
For example, the Summer Water Sign Cancer operates very

differently from the Winter Sign Pisces, because warm water in the summer and cold water in the winter are experienced very differently. That ocean you would happily play in during the Summer looks remarkably uninviting in the Winter. Each Sign of an Element is separated by 120 degrees. In Astrology this Aspect is called a Trine and it is considered a supportive, harmonious relationship.

The Fire Signs are Aries, Leo and Sagittarius. The Earth Signs are Taurus, Virgo and Capricorn. The Air Signs are Gemini, Libra and Aquarius. The Water Signs are Cancer, Scorpio and Pisces.

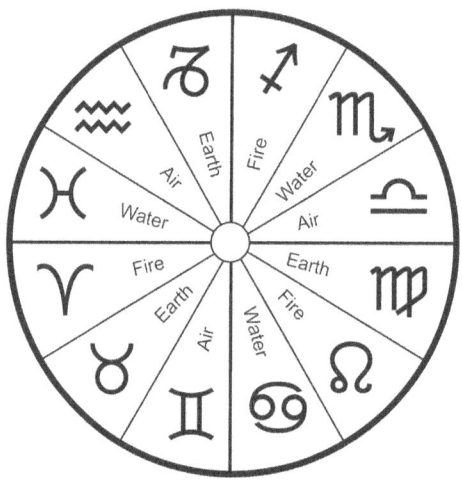

About the Chinese "Elements"

The concept of the Chinese 'Elements' has caused all kinds of confusion due to a mistranslation because the concept sounded similar, but the Western and Asian 'Elements' describe two different systems. As we stated, the Western system, which is also used by Indian Astrologers (Vedic) describes the States of Matter. The proper translation for the Chinese concept is 'Stages'. But please don't confuse that with the stages of the seasons that we just discussed. What the Chinese are talking about are the physiological actions of the Planets as described in the body.

This is a basic tenant of Chinese medicine. When you experience an event, physical, emotional or mental, it is processed by Planet after Planet, body system after system, until its influence on you is done. Most life events are handled routinely. But some events are traumatic, and that trip down the production line is rocky. That is why 'letting go' of an event is often the path to feeling better. Disease occurs when the event lands in one of those stages and gets stuck there.

Chinese medicine is about getting that process flowing again, by energizing or relaxing the correct body systems, and each relates to a Planet. There are five systems or stages; Metal (Mercury), Moon (Water), Wood (Saturn), Fire (Jupiter) and Earth (Venus). These are modulated by two qualities, Heart Warmth (Sun) and Hormonal Heat (Mars). That makes seven players; that is the same number as the traditional Western Planets that they describe. Read Chapter 15 to learn more about the Chinese approach to Astrology and healing.

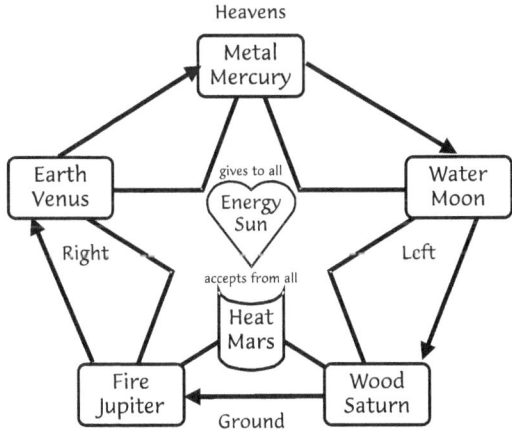

Fourth: What is their Quality? We can also define this as the Sign's 'standing' or 'positioning' because it is determined by the Sign's placement within its season. They are Cardinal, Fixed and Mutable. The Cardinal Signs are Aries, Cancer, Libra and Capricorn. The Fixed Signs are Taurus, Leo, Scorpio and Aquarius. The Mutable Signs are Gemini, Virgo, Sagittarius and Pisces.

The first 30 degrees of each season are the Cardinal Signs. They take action. The next 30 degrees are the Fixed Signs, they codify those actions into a system. The final 30 degrees are the Mutable Signs, that apply those actions and systems in human situations.

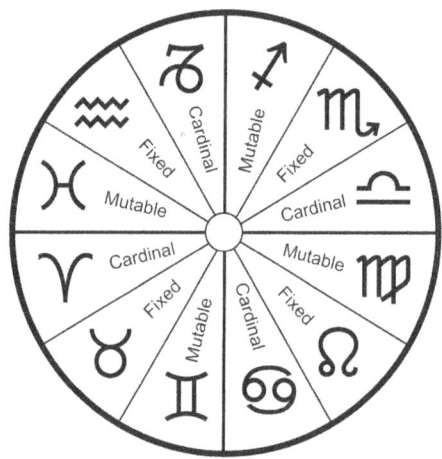

Then the next season begins with the next Cardinal Sign. Signs of the same Quality are separated from each other by either 90 or 180 degrees. Those "Aspects", the Square and Opposition, are considered challenging, but productive relationships. So, the Cardinal Sign Aries is 90 degrees from the Cardinal Signs Cancer and Capricorn, and 180 degrees from the Cardinal Signs Libra.
How the Sequence of the Signs Works

The 12 Signs make a sequential cycle that contains the three finer cycles. First: The Signs alternate from Dynamic to Receptive, starting with Dynamic Aries and ending with Receptive Pisces. Second: They start with the Fire Sign Aries to Earth Sign Taurus to Air Sign Gemini to Water Sign Cancer, then back to Fire Sign Leo and so on. Third: They start with the Cardinal Sign Aries, followed by Fixed Taurus and Mutable Gemini, then back to Cardinal Cancer and so on. These three imbedded cycles; Polarity, Element and Quality (or standing) tell you how the Signs act and how they relate to each other. This is important because life is all about roles and relationships!

What the Three Definitions Tell Us About the Signs

First: Signs of similar **Polarity** (Receptive or Dynamic) are mildly supportive of each other and are separated by multiples of 60 degrees. Example: The first degree of Dynamic Aries is 60 degrees from the first degree of the next Dynamic Sign Gemini. That Aspect, 60 degrees, is called a Sextile. Aries is a Fire Sign and Gemini is an Air Sign, so they are they both related to Father Sky. The next Sextile in the sequence, Receptive Earth Sign Taurus and Receptive Water Sign Cancer are both linked to Mother Earth.

Second: Signs of the same **Element** are very supportive of each other and connected by multiples of 120 degree, an Aspect called a Trine. Example: The first degree of the Air Sign Gemini is 120 degrees from the first degree of Air Signs Libra and Aquarius. In simplified Sun Sign Astrology people are often advised to find a partner in one of the other two related Element Signs. For example, a Virgo Sun should seek a Taurus or Capricorn Sun. As we said, relationships are everything.

In Chinese Astrology people are advised to find a mate four years older or younger than themselves. That is because their Jupiter positions will be in the same element, or Trine. For example, someone born in the Year of the Rabbit (Jupiter in Aries) should marry someone born in the Year or the Sheep (Jupiter in Leo) or the Year of the Pig (Jupiter in Sagittarius), the three Western Fire Signs. This promotes fiscal stability and mutual good luck. Sound advice!

Third: Signs having a similar **Quality** or Standing challenge each other to be productive and are connected by Aspects of 90 degrees (Square) and 180 degrees (Opposition). Example: The first degree of the Fixed Sign Taurus is 90 degrees from the first degrees of Leo and Aquarius and 180 degrees from the first degree of Scorpio.

Some Observations about the Seasons

In Western Astrology the year starts with Spring at the first degree of the Sign Aries. But, in Asia, the Springtime festival, called the Chinese New Year, begins at the New Moon in Aquarius, which can occur any time between the 19th of January and the 18th of February. That is where the concept of an early or late Spring comes from, that we celebrate on Groundhog Day. The Aquarius New Moon is when the energy of the Earth is drawn in.

In the northern hemisphere, it is after that New Moon when the seeds begin to stir in the moist, darkness of the Earth. Western Astrology, a Yang culture, prefers aggressive Aries as the starting point because that is when that new growth's red shoots burst into the light. Red is the color of the Planet Mars who rules Aries. Asia prefers Aquarius, a Sign that denies the ego in favor of the common good.

The 3 Signs of Spring: Aries, Taurus, Gemini

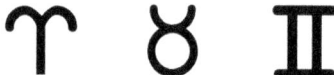

In Western Astrology the 3 Signs of Spring are Aries, when the first buds appear, **Taurus** when the green leaves unfurl and **Gemini** when the flying insects begin buzzing about spreading the pollen. **Aries** is a Dynamic, Cardinal Fire Sign ruled by Mars and symbolized by the Ram, because it is an impetuous, lustful time of year. **Taurus** is a Receptive, Fixed Earth Sign ruled by Venus and symbolized by the Bull (although a Cow is a better description since it is a Receptive Sign) because it is patient and stable.

Gemini is a Dynamic, Mutable Air Sign ruled by Mercury and symbolized by the Twins. It is associated with the twin brothers, Romulus and Remus, who established Rome and were known for their joint talents of enterprise and mischief.

The 3 Signs of Summer: Cancer, Leo, Virgo

♋ ♌ ♍

The first day of Summer begins with Cancer, a Receptive, Cardinal Water Sign ruled by the Moon, symbolized by the Crab and associated with the sea, the tides, the Mother and the home-life. The Sign is closely associated with mothering and the first nurturing liquid the child experiences, the maternal milk. This is the season when the flowers turn into the first edible fruits.

That is followed by Leo, a Dynamic, Fixed Fire Sign ruled by the Sun and symbolized by the Lion, the King of the Jungle. Now the trees are filled with fruit for the picking and there is an abundance of flowers for both vitamins and matters of the heart. These first two Signs relate to the high Summer when the living is easy, and people go on vacation.

The third Summer Sign is Virgo, a Receptive, Mutable, Earth Sign ruled by Mercury and symbolized by the Virgin. Virgo is the largest stellar constellation and before the Christian Era these Stars were known as the 'Great Goddess'. This is harvest time and Virgo's legendary industriousness, attention to detail and cleanliness describes the diligent efforts of gathering and sorting fruit, vegetables, grains and winemaking.

History says that it was women who led humanity from the hunter gatherer life to agriculture, by cultivating storable grains and grasses at the riversides. Virgo is when the family and the community work together quickly and efficiently, to bring in the grapes for wine and the grains and beans as staples to last them through the Winter.

Because girls mature faster than boys and often have better dexterity, their contribution was especially prized at the close of Summer, when harvest requires patient, skilled hands.

The 3 Signs of Autumn: Libra, Scorpio, Sagittarius

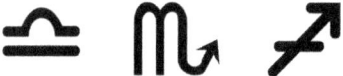

The first day of Autumn begins with Libra, a Dynamic, Cardinal Air Sign ruled by Venus and symbolized by the Scales. It is related to partnerships and marriage because this is when each family's seasonal contribution and share is carefully and fairly measured on the scales.

As the leaves disappear and the first Signs of Winter make their appearance **Scorpio begins**, a Receptive, Fixed, Water Sign ruled by Mars and symbolized by the Scorpion, although it is alternately symbolized by the Snake, the Eagle and the Phoenix.

It traditionally relates to the cooperative use of power. As the rains bring the harvest to a close and the leaves fall away serious, private tasks are required with the approaching Winter, so the bargaining gets tougher and secrets more vital. The hard frosts set in at higher elevations and the first ice, or Fixed Water, appears on the ponds.

As the last leaves are gone **Sagittarius** begins, a Dynamic, Mutable, Fire Sign ruled by giant Jupiter and symbolized by the Centaur Archer. This is the time when the views expand with the first frosts, the protective cover of leaves is gone, and the hunters venture out.

With a patron like Zeus, aka the 'Big Guy in the Plaid Suit', for his wonderfully colorful, swirling surface, it is unsurprising that 'Sag' is known for optimism, philosophy, travel and entrepreneurship.

The 3 Signs of Winter: Capricorn, Aquarius, Pisces

The first day of Winter begins with Capricorn, a Receptive, Cardinal, Earth Sign ruled by Saturn and symbolized by the Sea Goat, a Goat with the tail of a Fish. Traditionally it relates to time and maturity. Where Sagittarius expands, Capricorn contracts. This is when Winter sets in seriously, everything contracts with the cold and wood is brought in to fuel the fire. It is a Sign that deals with prestige because the success of the year's efforts will show in the quality of the winter coats you and your family are wearing at the Winter Solstice Festival.

As Winter deepens, **Aquarius** begins, a Dynamic, Fixed, Air Sign also ruled by Saturn and symbolized by the Water Bearer, although some experts say it is the Water Pourer. The symbol relates to the innovation of irrigation at the beginning of the agricultural era. This is the time of year when rice farmers drain and repair their growing ponds. Aquarius is about community action for the common good, your social connections and friendships. It describes the community that your history and efforts have given you access to.

Winter ends with **Pisces**, a Receptive, Mutable, Water Sign ruled by Jupiter and symbolized by Two Fishes, one swimming towards the deep and another swimming towards the light. In Pisces Winter begins to lose its grip, the hard ground is thawing, the melting snow softens the seeds helping their germination. The hint of Spring is bringing hope as is suitable for a Sign ruled by expansive Jupiter. With the completion of Pisces, we find ourselves once again hopefully approaching the first day of Spring and the new cycle.

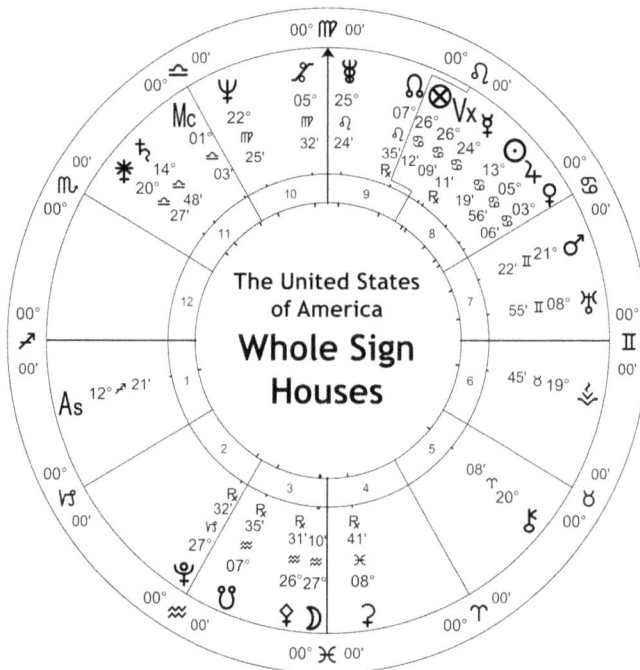

Placidus Moves the Sun from the 8th to the 7th House

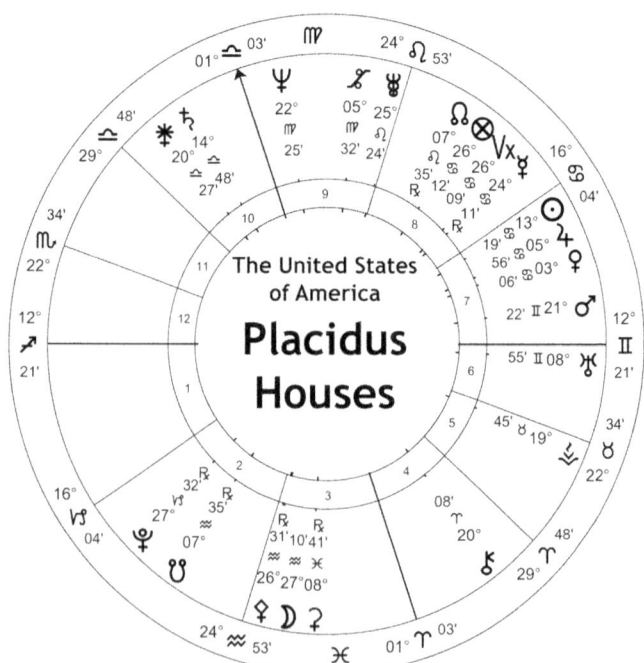

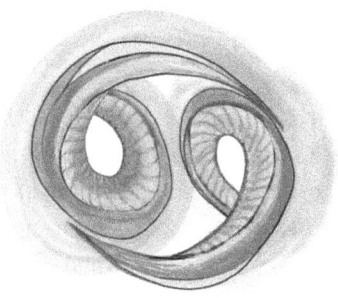

Chapter Four: The Whole Sign House System

There are numerous House systems that have been developed by mathematicians over the centuries. The one an Astrologer uses is usually based on what they were taught. We have used many different ones, but over the years we found that the Whole Sign House system, which is the most ancient and traditional, worked best in our specialties of health and location, which are practical, well-grounded studies.

There are two reasons for the proliferation of systems. **First**, over the centuries, Astrological knowledge was poorly preserved and mis-translated from the ancient Greek, Latin, Aramaic and Chinese. This led to erroneous information, confusion and problems that led mathematicians to seek solutions.

Second, there are two major House based Astrology systems; Western (European) and Vedic (Indian). They each developed their own systems, while Chinese Astrology was conceived on a different, Imperial premise.

We are going to discuss the Western variations. Three of the most popular Western House Systems are Placidus, Koch and Whole Sign. The first two vary from the Whole Sign Houses primarily by starting the First and Seventh Houses at the degrees of the Ascendant and Descendant. They also start the Tenth and Fourth Houses at the Midheaven and IC. The Cusps (The first degree of a Sign or House) of the other Houses vary and rarely start at the beginning of a Sign.

That means that Signs can span two Houses and other Signs can be enclosed in Houses with no connection to the Cusps (called Intercepted). Since the Signs commanding the Cusps tell us which Bodies hold sway over these regions of the life, with unequal Houses, some Signs get greater regions of control while others get short changed. Philosophically, we have a hard time thinking that any Celestial Body is willing to stand around with a cork in its mouth when it comes to having a say about that Chart's direction. On the other hand, for the sensitive, mentally quick, creative practitioner, these wandering Cusps open an array of timely nuanced interpretation possibilities.

For us, working with health and location, they open a few too many! For instance, these wandering Cusps can take two Planets next to each other in the same Sign (Conjunct) and place them in two different Houses, or arenas. Clearly those Celestial Bodies are on the same team, but a mathematical calculation says they are playing on two different fields. That's like saying that two teammates, wearing the same uniform, are being told to play two different sports; Karen is playing basketball, but her teammate Susan was sent to help the debating team! Astrology reflects life, *"As Above So Below"* and dividing Conjunct Planets into different Houses is a wacky style of coaching.

The ancient Astrologers did not differentiate between the meanings of the Signs and the Houses, but they applied them differently: The Signs describe time, while the Houses describe location and physical space, and the Celestial Bodies are the players crisscrossing the field. Compared to the other systems, Whole Sign is wonderfully simple which is nice since very little in Celestial mechanics is simple.

In Whole Signs, the First House is the entire 30 degrees of the Rising Sign. The Ascendant is a specific degree inside the First

House. The opposing point, or Descendant, is a specific degree inside the Seventh House.

Using Whole Signs, the Fourth House of home is the Fourth Sign counting from the First House, or the Rising. The Tenth House of career is the Tenth Sign as counted from the First House, or the Rising. The Midheaven, describing the spot directly above your head on the Ecliptic, can now appear in the Ninth, Tenth or Eleventh Houses. The opposite spot below you on the Ecliptic, the IC or "Imum Coeli", can be in the Third, Fourth or Fifth Houses.

The placement of the Midheaven and IC in those varied Houses shows the focus of the native's career and home life. These four angles are pointers. The Ascendant describes the Self, where the Descendant, the opposite point on the Ecliptic, is about their partner. At the top of the Chart, the Midheaven or MC, is the 'flag above your castle' while the opposite IC represents your core family and home life, your foundation. The MC is noticed more because it is out there in the world. The IC is more instinctive, like the way the aroma of your mother's chicken soup makes you feel at home.

When the MC is in the Ninth House the career tilts towards being an expert or professional, including educators, physicians, attorneys, accountants, consultants, pilots and astrologers, etc.

The MC in the Tenth House reveals people who seek prominence in their community. They tend to have a balanced career where they are involved in all aspects of their work. This is like the person who faces their desk directly at the door with access on both sides, so they can reach out with both sides of their personality.

The MC in the Eleventh House is for people who are involved in their community and who like the business side of business. In other words, they are less concerned with career acclaim and more interested in the bottom line. They also work through non-profits and public service, where the ego satisfaction is less important than the sense of shared accomplishment.

Having the IC in the Third, Fourth or Fifth Houses changes the part of the family life where they are most comfortable. In the Third House the relationship and communication with the siblings, cousins and peers matters most. They tend to remain close to the 'kids' they grew up with and want to light heartedly explore the world of the MC in the Ninth House. The IC in the Fourth House shows a person who is anchored in their heritage.

They look at their parents, grandparents and great grandparents, and so on, as the authority, by example, that defines their values. Their commitment to continuity is expressed in the tenacity of the MC in the Tenth House. When the IC is in the Fifth House it is the creativity of their home life that gives them joy.

That experience is what allows them to comfortably navigate the inventive chaos of the MC in the Eleventh House. The IC and MC exist synergistically and Celestial bodies near one affect the other.

Now that you have a sense of why we use Whole Sign Houses, we suggest you try it out. It is remarkably easy to use.

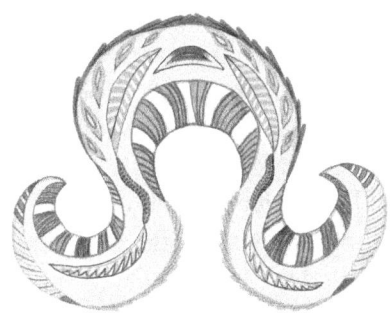

Chapter Five: The Houses as Place

Note, in case you skipped the previous chapter: The ancient Astrologers didn't differentiate between the Signs and Houses, probably because the approach was so location-based. In the interim many House systems have been developed. As we explained in detail in the previous chapter, we use the Whole Sign House System which is most similar to the ancient approach.

The Houses and the Angles

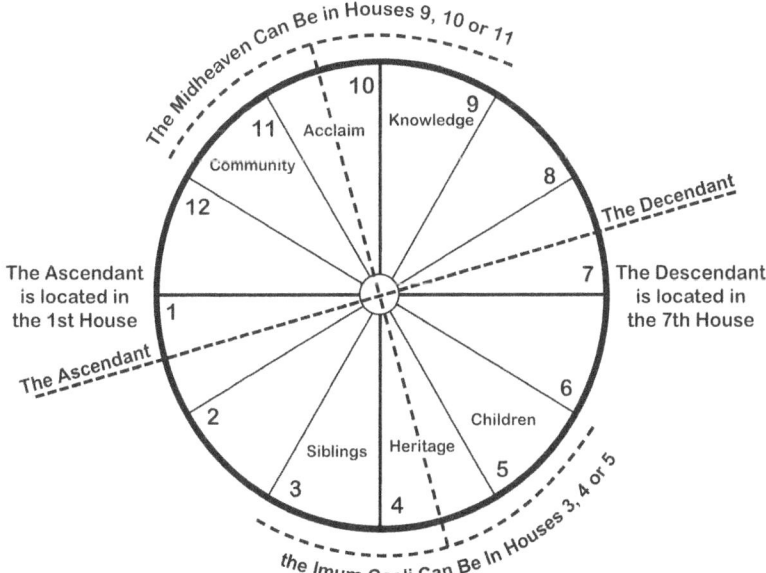

The third component of an Astrological Chart is the System of Houses where we bring everything down to Earth. The twelve Houses start in the left and run counterclockwise. The Houses take the positions of the celestial Bodies above and relate them to your physical location here in Earth. The Houses personalize the information for the 'Native', which is the Astrological term for the person for whom the Natal Chart is calculated. A Chart Cast for an event is called an Elective Chart.

A Chart is a specialized map and the Houses tell you the compass directions to generally face to find that Planet in the sky. Ancient Astrologers called the sky the forehead of God and Astrology was their way of reading those celestial thoughts, which offers a whole new perspective about the art of face reading! A very useful skill!

Like the Signs, the Houses divide the space around the native, or event's location into twelve segments, but while the Signs are sky based, the Houses are Earth based. The meanings of the Houses are related to the Twelve Signs, but the Signs are about actions, while the Houses are about the arenas where those actions happen. The House angles relate to compass directions. But, because the players in this game are the Sun, Moon and Planets, the Chart is focused on where they travel. That path is called the Ecliptic and in the Northern Hemisphere that is towards the Southern Sky.

The Chart most Astrologers use is not a compass rose, but a picture of the Earth and Sky from your point of view. To the left is the East and the right is the West. But, the two important points are the Ascendant and the Descendant. These are the spots where the Ecliptic intersects the horizon to the East and West, or where the Sun would rise (Ascend), and set (Descend). In the Northern Hemisphere these are to the Southeast and Southwest. The top of the Chart is the sky above and that is called the Midheaven, or MC. It is the spot on the Ecliptic directly towards the South. The bottom of the Chart is the sky below and the point opposite the MC is called the "Imum Coeli" or IC. Now that we have our bearings, let's look at the meanings of the Houses.

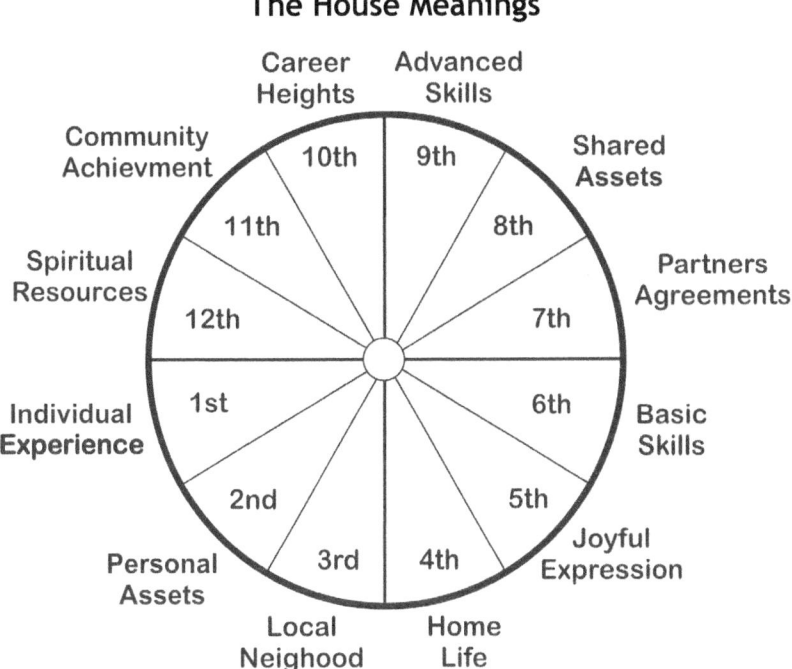

Life is complex, and it has many arenas in which we operate. Consider for a moment all the ways that you define yourself: Child, grandchild, sibling, cousin, heritage, race, genetics, spouse, parent, friend, employee, employer, member, citizen, artist, professional, Sun Sign, ethnicity, religion, belief, politics, sexual orientation, blood type, diet preferences and personality types, etc. The Houses divide these various roles into twelve sections. You can imagine them as twelve places where you live your life.

The First House is where you were born. The **Second** is where you keep your treasured possessions. The **Third** is where you read and write. The **Fourth** is where you cook. The **Fifth** is where you play and make love. The **Sixth** is where you use a marketable skill and care for others. The **Seventh** is where you marry and make commitments. The **Eighth** is where you share your marriage bed, your body and your bank account. The **Ninth** is where you live in a foreign land and use a foreign or professional language. The **Tenth** is where you work and attain your reputation. The **Eleventh** is where you meet with friends to accomplish things together. The **Twelfth** is where you meet with your divine community.

When a Celestial Body is in one of those Houses it is most active in that area of life. A concentration of Planets in a House shows a great deal of activity in that area, a focused perspective and often a talent or skill that you bring to the game. For example, when a person has the Sun and several positively connected Planets in the Fourth House, which is associated with the Home and Family Life, a large percentage of their satisfaction and fulfillment will come from there. Their point of view will be strongly influenced by the family heritage.

An empty House doesn't mean that part of your life is devoid of activity, because the Sign residing in the House shows which Celestial Body rules that House. Who is the landlord? Example: If the Sign in the House is Gemini or Virgo then Mercury Rules the House, even if it is in a different House. When the ruling Celestial Body is well connected, that arena it Rules can see significant activity. For example, if you don't have any Planets in the 7th House of marriage, but have Taurus ruling the House, putting Venus in charge, and Venus is in the Sign Libra, its Dynamic Ruling Sign, you can figure marriage and partnership will be a Significant part of your life.

The First House starts in the East and it contains the Ascendant, or Rising Sign, which is one of the big three indicators that most people know about their Charts, along with the positions of the Sun and Moon. The Ascendant and the Planets in the First House describe your physical body, general appearance, personal outlook and how you encounter the world. It is also how people see you! When you wake up in the morning and your eyes pop open, that moment is the Ascendant, conscious of being incarnate in this world. When a client doesn't know their birth-time, a critical factor in calculating an accurate Chart, we consider what Sign and Planets most closely describes their physical appearance. There is a good chance they are in the First House, which allows us to correct the Chart's time somewhat.

For some general examples; red haired people often have one of the three Fire Signs Rising, Aries, Leo or Sagittarius. A softer, rounder appearance often reveals a Water Sign rising, Cancer, Scorpio or Pisces. Capricorn and Aquarius Rising, both Saturn ruled Signs, often bestow high cheek bones and a prominent bone structure, because the Ruling Planet Saturn rules the skeletal system. A spike of white hair along the brow often shows up with Scorpio Rising.

The Houses are divided into four quadrants, 1,2 & 3. Then 4, 5 & 6. Then 7, 8 & 9. Then 10, 11 & 12. These have their own positioning terms. The first House in the sequence is Angular, the second is Succedent, the third is Cadent. The Angular House is where actions are initiated. The Succedent House is where the actions started in the Angular House are made part of a system, securing its place in society. In the Cadent House is where that codified knowledge is applied to people. This is related to the concept of Cardinal, Fixed and Mutable, but applied to locations instead of activities.

The Personal Houses, 1 through 6

The first six Houses span the lower half of the Chart. They represent the personal life, starting with the 1) personal self and body, 2) the personal possessions, 3) the local neighborhood, 4) the home, 5) the place of joy and expression and finally 6) the place where one learns skills. With the Seventh House the Chart ventures into the social, public world.

The First House, which contains the Ascendant, starts the sequence and runs counterclockwise for thirty degrees. There is an obvious correlation between the 12 Houses and the 12 Signs, with Aries, Ruled by Mars, being the most related to the First, an Angular House, and the location of the Ascendant. People with numerous Planets in the First House are good at encountering new people and situations. They bring a great deal of energy to their personal expression.

Agressive and engaging salespeople often have numerous strong Planets in the First House, close to the Ascendant. Don't underestimate the importance of the Angles. When Planets are within 10 degrees, to either side, of the Ascendant or Midheaven, they have more leverage. Since the First House relates to the individual, the newborn, the protean self, then it makes sense that the Second House relates to those gifts which they are given by nature and family.

The Second House is associated with the Sign Taurus, the Bull, Ruled by Venus and that which we possess personally. It is a Succedent House. Those 'possessions' start with innate strengths that are theirs alone, natural talents and beauty, the sound of their voice, the senses of taste and smell, love and food. As life goes on it relates to the arts, music, clothes, money and real estate.

The Sign in the Second House tells you which Planet commands the House, so the condition, or strength of that Planet will tell you how well-endowed that native is with these talents. The Planets inside the House highlight skill sets they use in that arena. For example, since the Second House is most related to Taurus, which is ruled by Venus, if you have Venus in that House, in any Sign, it empowers both the House and the Planet by the power of strategic positioning.

In the Third House you now have a possession and your sibling or cousin has something you want, so you make a deal, you 'play ball', you interact. The Third House is most associated with the Sign Gemini, the Twins, Ruled by Mercury. It is about social interchange. It is a Cadent House. This is where the child learns to speak so the Third House is about all kinds of communication, especially among those close to you. It relates to mobility and short distance travel, the neighborhood, the places where people know you because you are somebody's child. As an adult this applies to people you see in your everyday experience.

Also, because the Second House deals with your natural beauty and attractiveness and the Third House is about interaction and language, it is also the place where flirting skills are developed, so it includes the playfulness of language. The condition of the Planet ruling the Third House tells you a great deal about how you speak, including your accent. The Planets inside the House will color the style in which you communicate. For instance, Jupiter, the expander, strongly placed in the Third House can give a person a tendency to be loud and expressive in speech, but also show a talent for foreign languages.

The Fourth House sits at the base of the Chart and it is the foundation of your life, your home, family and parents. It is associated with the Sign Cancer, the Crab, which is ruled by the Moon, who is associated with the Mother and the matriarchal line. It is an Angular House, which is not surprising since the Mother initiates numerous actions in a child's life. That includes the way in which the home is chosen and arranged and the types of foods and smells that are passed down through the women in your life.

The Sign commanding the House and the Planets there describe your early home life, and the type of home you will make for yourself. This is a place where emotions live, sensitivity, receptivity and soul nourishment. It shows how intuitive, emotionally flexible and resilient you are in family situations. It is helpful to remember that the Moon is the fastest of the Celestial Bodies, covering a Sign in two and a half days.

While we tend to see the Fourth House as our foundation, it is as much about emotional foundations as physical. The other Earthly foundations are found in the Second House where the related Receptive Sign, Taurus, has four hooves firmly grounded on the Earth. Surprisingly, having the Moon in the Fourth House, rather than showing a tendency to stay put, because of that mobility, shows a person who is inclined to change residences, rearrange the furniture, consider new homes and in all ways express the Moon's high rate of speed. The state of the Fourth House, along with the Sign of the Moon, shows the kind of nurturing environment a person creates.

The Fifth House. If the Fourth House is where nest building takes place, the Fifth is where the child in introduced, and the traditional descriptor of this House is Children. It is a Succedent House, and relates to Leo, the Lion, Ruled by the Sun and associated with the King or Queen. Beyond children the Fifth House relates to romance and creative expressions, whether it is art, crafts, business or games. Even though the Second House has a strong connection to the arts, the Fifth House is about the enthusiasm and creativity that goes into making something new.

The Sun rules the heart and any activity that comes from the heart plays out in the Fifth House. While the Third House is where the art of flirting is first developed, the Fifth House is where that flirting is put to good use, so the love life is connected to this area. The Planets ruling the House will tell you who you find attractive. While the Seventh House better describes what you look for in a mate, the Fifth House says what you look for in a lover.

For example, if you have Gemini in the Fifth House you might be attracted to 'bad boys' or 'bad girls', youthful, impish and playful. But in the Leo ruled Seventh House you will tend to look for a mate who is Leonine, commanding, heart based and romantic. If you find someone with Gemini Rising and a Leo Sun, you could get the best of both worlds.

The Sixth House. The romance of the Fifth House will eventually lead to marriage in the Seventh House, but first it needs to go through some refinement, namely the fiery forge of the Sixth House. This is a Cadent House related to Virgo, Ruled by Mercury. If that controlled, forceful imagery seems out of character for the starry-eyed Virgin, consider that her alter ego is Vulcan, the blacksmith God who works that forge.

With the Sixth House we enter an interesting territory. As we've gone through the Houses, each has related to a specific Sign which is ruled by a Planet. As we venture on the other side of Leo, we come to the first House where the Planet Rulerships repeat. That is because Gemini and the Third House, and Virgo and the Sixth House are both Ruled by Mercury. Both Houses relate to basic skills, the Third to language and the Sixth House to the physical dexterity and logical thought needed to accomplish useful, everyday tasks. These are the kind of activities you do in your daily work, either at home or your workplace. It is often repetitive, but requires experience, hand eye coordination, muscle memory, attention to detail and endurance to accomplish.

The connection here to Virgo, the young woman is not surprising, because women often fill these roles. These are the activities that ensure the health and wellbeing of the people in your life. These include cleaning, cooking, sorting, preserving, building, repairing and recording information. Traditionally, this is the province of craftspeople, tradespeople, nurses, cooks, maids and there is a workaday, unpretentious feeling about the Sixth House.

The Sign at the Cusp and the Planets inside often reveal the state of health you will enjoy. As a person considers who they will marry, the Sixth House is where the Father of the Bride wants to know what kind of work this young man does, and the Mother of the potential Groom wants to know if this young lady can cook and sew? Admittedly, this description is old school, and the skill sets required of modern women and men to support a good relationship have changed, but they need to compliment and overlap, so the couple can cooperate and keep themselves safe and sound. The Sixth House is about the basic skills that support your wellbeing, as well as being helpful to your family, including learning marketable skills.

The Social Houses

The Seventh House is where we venture above the Horizon for the first time, moving from the personal world, represented by the First House through the Sixth, into the social world of Houses Seven through Twelve. The Seventh House is Angular, the location of the Descendant, related to Libra and Ruled by Venus.

It is the place where agreements, contracts and marriages are sealed. You've met the person who makes your heart sing in the Fifth House. You've met each other's parents and gained approval in the Sixth House. Up to now the love affair has been private, but now you've gotten a license at the court House, and you are standing up in front of society, everyone who is important to you, committing to a social, legal relationship that extends beyond yourself. That relationship will be regulated by rules not of your making.

The Seventh House is the Dynamic side of Venus, who rules Libra. It is formal but graceful, patient but fair, carefully negotiated, with the goal of welding partners together, in consideration of the practical issues involved when sharing responsibilities with another person. This careful dance is not any different from the myriad contracts people commit to daily in modern life.

When people click the accept box on a computer screen, making a purchase, they haven't carefully considered what they are getting into. That is why companies make a big deal about being transparent, to remove the fear that accompanies purchases. The Seventh House, as one of the upper Houses, is connected to the sky above and the Descendant is where the Sun sets. It is the place where people come together with those they trust for food and warmth during the night. There are few times when a person feels as forlorn as when the Sun is setting, and they have no place to find comfort. The Seventh is a serious House, a place of commitment, where people become part of something larger than themselves, opening them to greater possibilities found in the ensuing Houses.

The Eighth House. This is a Succedent House most related to Scorpio, the Receptive Sign Ruled by Mars. It is where guidelines are established for cooperation. The traditional description for the Eighth House is downright dire; transformational experiences, birth, death and inheritance! Really?

That doesn't tell us much, so let's flesh that out, because the Eighth House is a powerful place where people share responsibility and secrets. That focus on the end of life for this House came out of historic short life spans, and high birth mortality. Marriages were often short-lived due to the dangers of childbirth, physical work, hunting and war.

The House is better called the place of legal inheritance and legacy because it deals with the delegation of assets related to those partnerships formed in the Seventh.

The Eighth is the polarity of the Second House, which deals with personal possessions. In comparison, the Eighth House deals with shared Possessions. The ruling Planet of the House and the Planets inside give you an idea of how the native handles power and resources, for which they share responsibility or ownership.

The House will often see Transits when the person is dealing with inheritance issues. A person's own time of passing rarely shows up there. More often it shows up in the Charts of the people connected to them as they deal with that legacy.

About How the 'Social' 9th, 10th & 11th Houses Work

The Houses run counterclockwise, so each House contributes to the following. They also provide special support for those they are related to by polarity and especially Element. The Tenth is supported by the Sixth House by a Trine (A supportive aspect or relationship of 120 degrees), so the basic working skills developed in the Sixth support your attainment in the Tenth House.

The Tenth House, in turn, supports through a Trine, the Second House of personal possessions. So, the career achievement in the Tenth contributes to your personal gain in terms of beauty, comfort and security. This supportive relationship is essential to these three, socially dependent career Houses (9, 10 & 11) at the top of the Chart. Those three Houses are the definition of 'reputation'.

The Ninth House. This is a Cadent House most related to Sagittarius, the Dynamic Sign of Jupiter, the largest of the Planets. The shared power from the preceding two Houses is now entering practical application in people's lives. The traditional description of the Ninth House is the word 'Fortune', so its reputation as lucky is long-standing. It relates to higher education, long-distance travel, and the benefits from professional help and benefactors. It is the space of professors, professionals, entrepreneurs, import and exports, foreign languages, philosophy and formal religion.

Here is where one expands their horizons, they take a chance, they consider ideas and philosophies from cultures they encounter in their explorations. The first time that a person lives far from their family is often for school or work. In the opposite Third House one learns what linguists call the 'milk language'.

The Ninth House is where they learn not only foreign languages, but the arcane languages of their profession; medicine, law, business or philosophy. In the early 1800's there were no institutions for higher learning in the Americas, so young people risked their lives on sailing ships to live in Paris, where Universities were free to foreigners. There was one catch, courses in medicine, law or art were taught in French, the international language. The result was a generation of North and South American professors, professionals and artists who were accustomed to reading French books and papers for the rest of their professional lives.

This created a linguistic wall, often made higher by the requirements of Latin and Greek, between them and the common folk, a cultural ivory tower that the professions dwelled within for many years. That is the nature of the Ninth House; the specialized knowledge that sets you apart and makes you valuable to the wider society that is represented by the upper part of the Chart. The Sign and Planets describe the 'elevated view' that will carry throughout your life.

The Tenth is an Angular House related to Capricorn, the Receptive Sign of Saturn. It is where you, now enriched by travel and education, assume your position, however junior, in your chosen field. If the Ninth House is the time of jeans and back packs, the Tenth House is the time for business suits and briefcases. Capricorn is often depicted as serious and masculine, the father figure. But, while maturity is a hallmark of Saturn, it is important to remember that Capricorn is a Receptive Sign. I prefer to imagine Capricorn as a grove of giant Redwood trees that are connected through a wide network of roots. This would describe a business person's love of skyscrapers.

This also describes how mature women, who stay in an area, develop extensive social connections in their communities. That's why the most successful, sustainable companies have large numbers of women working there for long periods of time.

Their talent for networking and a tendency to be risk averse helps them build in consistent, enduring ways, the way a family is made. Within the three phases of career (The Ninth, Tenth and Eleventh Houses) the Tenth is where people make the greatest amount of progress towards personal reputation. The Ninth House experience of school and travel is often expensive while the Eleventh House is where people share their wealth with their community. But in the Tenth House people work because they are being paid and they seek opportunities to improve their status so they can increase their income. The Sign and Planets in the Tenth House tell you how a person conducts this stage of their career.

The Midheaven and Career

There is a helpful indicator of career that is only found when you use the Whole Sign House System. In the popular Placidus or Koch House systems the Midheaven defines the Cusp of the Tenth House. But in Whole Signs the Midheaven does not! Instead, in the temperate latitudes the Midheaven can be found inside any of the three career Houses, Ninth, Tenth and Eleventh. In the extreme latitudes the MC can be found even further afield, saying much about those who choose to live in extreme weather conditions. Read our detailed explanation of Whole Sign Houses in the next section.

Think of the Midheaven as the flag above your castle, it signals your position in society to the world. The House where the Midheaven appears, flying that flag, is often the primary focus of the career. In judging that, don't forget that the other two Houses also affect social standing. If they contain powerful career Planets those Houses will be active areas.

For example, you could have the Midheaven in the Eleventh House, but have Saturn in the Tenth House or Jupiter in the Ninth, both powerful through strategic position. There would no denying those hefty influences in the person's life and their career focus would likely span Houses, a common experience among business owners, entrepreneurs and artists, who must play multiple roles equally well.

The Eleventh is a Succedent House, associated with Aquarius, the Dynamic Sign of Saturn. It is where the actions taken in the Tenth, are systemized into working and social groups that provide sustaining structures, or networks. The Eleventh is why people will stay in jobs where the work is not fulfilling, but their personal interaction with co-workers and customers is enriching. The Tenth and Eleventh Houses are the region of Saturn, where the needs of the ego are sublimated for the sake of the group and long-term action and results are the goal.

That is why, within industries and professions, social organizations bring people with similar ideas and issues together to exchange information and socialize. Fraternal groups, churches, clubs are all types of assemblies that allow people to satisfy that very human need for companionship. They cooperate on missions that are beyond their individual capabilities. That personal satisfaction exceeds the small amount of contribution each person makes.

This social arena, the chaos and genius marketplace and the workplace, the cooperation of friends and community, is the province of the Eleventh House. While this has an altruistic flavor, there is a business side to this House, because people prefer to do business with people they know and like. Being connected to a large social organization encourages your community to bring their business to your door. The Eleventh House is an expression of the saying, *"It's not what you know, but who you know that makes your money"*.

The Eleventh House has a reputation for innovation because original ideas come out of social interaction among people with intersecting expertise, where the free exchange of ideas among equals stimulates creative problem solving. When one person can raise the issue, several others may offer solutions and sometimes the synthesis provides a better solution than the individual expert. The Eleventh House goal is avoiding problems in the future. That's why professional Astrologers often have a strong focus in the Eleventh House and Mercury, the Planet most associated with divination, aka seeing the future.

It is helpful to recognize that Aquarius, depicted as the Water Bearer or Pourer and associated with the Eleventh House, is one the three Human Signs, the others being Gemini, the Twins and Virgo the Virgin. All three are social, highly communicative Signs that represent the three strongest Signs of Mercury. Virgo is the Receptive Ruler. Gemini is the Dynamic Ruler and Aquarius is the Exalted Sign which means it is the ultimate insider. So, Mercury in Aquarius possesses special leverage and influence in areas of communication and social interaction. It possesses a unique ability to connect multiple energies together to accomplish the task at hand. The image of the Water Pourer symbolizes the person irrigating plants, a task essential for building a stable community, as compared to a nomadic tribe.

The Twelfth is a Cadent House most connected to Pisces, the Receptive Sign of Jupiter. The traditional descriptors for the Twelfth House include the words prison, hospital, monastery and places of restriction. Not the most inspiring image for a very special House. That image comes from a time when life spans were shorter and there were no social security nets, so debtor's prison was a common part of people's lives. In a current sense the Twelfth House, in its sequence of life, represents a time when people are restricted by dwindling finances or failing health. Historically wealthy people often left public life in their later years and entered a monastery or convent to spend their final years in devotion and service, but there is much more to it than that.

The Twelfth House is considered a place of retreat from the world, but it is active throughout your life. Every time you meditate or participate in a spiritual or religious ritual you are in the Twelfth House. For many artists, the studio is their place of refuge where they connect with their imagination and the divine energies. It is the place of dreams and imagination, so in this time when movies and storytelling have become such a prevalent part of our lives, the Twelfth, like the innovative Eleventh House, have become much busier places for people to occupy. This expansion fits in well with the following ideas.

The discoveries of Uranus and Neptune, which Astrologers feel are associated on a higher frequency with Aquarius and Pisces, has changed the interpretations of the Eleventh and Twelfth Houses. By becoming aware of these 'invisible' Planets, modern society has changed their experience of those parts of life outside the walls of Saturn. There is a greater fascination with inventors and outlaws, associated with the Eleventh House, as well as drugs, spiritual pursuits and manufactured realities, related to the Twelfth House.

Where the Eleventh House and Aquarius have been associated with the technological revolution, the Twelfth House and Pisces is associated with spirituality, inspiration, creativity and the artistry of illusion that we find in our movies and other technologies. Artists often have very strong Planets in their Twelfth Houses because the studio is a safe, inspired place away from the world.

It is helpful to recall that Pisces is the Receptive Sign of Jupiter, a Planet that relates to travel and faraway places, especially when that faraway place is in the imagination or the dream state. Many of the Significant spiritual teachings have come to the West from faraway Asia and India. Spiritual seekers are often travelers. The common Italian name Pellegrino means Pilgrim. Making a pilgrimage to Jerusalem or a Haj to Mecca are significant events in a devotee's life.

The Twelfth House is the end of the cycle started in the First House and Aries, where the ego first declares itself, "I am". Descartes's declaration "I think therefore I am" is a Third House statement, as the person moves beyond the instinctual experience of the First and Second Houses and develops their intellect. When Popeye said, "I am what I am and dat's all what I am", that was probably a Sixth House statement. It is the virgin, pure human free of anything else. When you ask, "You are what you are, but what have you done for me lately?", you are coming from the Eighth House, where people jockey for power.

In the process of dissolving the old self the Twelfth House is a place for preparing the ground for the next evolution, represented by the First House. In the temperate Northern Hemisphere, during the period which Pisces spans from late February to late March, Winter is ending, and the resources of the past year break down and become the disorganized nutrients for the new seeds. That may be why the Twelfth House often has a sense of disarray, like the artist's studio. Picasso would never let anyone clean his studio. He insisted that the dust be left untouched for fear of disrupting the creative connection.

The adventurous actions of career initiated in the Ninth, then crystallized in the Tenth House and systemized in the Eleventh now enter a time of reflection, when the native considers how their actions and decisions connected them to their world, for better or worse. The twelfth House is the place of regrets, forgiveness and dreams, but it contains within it the seeds of hope for the future. The Sign commanding the House and the Planets within show how you access your spiritual resources, through imagination, meditation, music, artwork and devotion.

This chapter sums up the three main components, Planets, Signs and Houses, that are the foundation upon which everything else built. Next, we will explain how the relationship between the Planets, through the Planetary Rulers and Dignities, which is essential to understanding how the Aspects work, which will come next. These are many other nuances in an Astrological Chart, but these three parts that we covered so far are the essential alphabet.

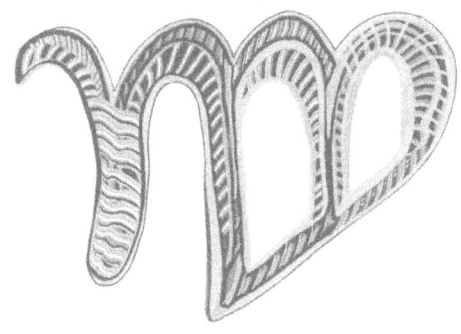

Chapter Six: Traditional Versus Modern Planetary Rulers

Understanding how the Planets and Signs are related is key to understanding how a Chart works. Their 'family tree' is called the Table of Dignities, an ancient system that shows the connections between the seven visible Celestial bodies and the twelve Signs. That's where the term, 'Planetary Ruler' comes from, as in, 'the Moon Rules Cancer'. On a family tree, a person can have multiple connections that determine their role. They may be listed as a child, sibling, cousin, spouse, parent or grandparent. In a similar way, each 'Planet' is connected to six Signs, filling a different role in each. Another way to think of a Planet is as an actor that dresses in varied costumes to play distinctly different roles on the stage.

Before we return to the Rulers and the Table of Dignities in the next chapter, we need to clear up some confusion. The Table Astrologers have used for thousands of years was seriously disrupted when Uranus was discovered in the 1700's, followed by Neptune the 1800's and Pluto in the 1900's. Their appearance threw a 'boomerang into the knitting' and it spurred contemporary Astrologers' misguided attempts to jam these new Planets into the ancient Table. They took 'Ruling Signs' away from the original Planets and gave them to the newcomers, oblivious to the other relationships on the family tree.

They forgot about the Law of Polarity, which explains why each Planet has two 'Ruling' Signs, one Feminine (Receptive) and another Masculine (Dynamic), like Mercury who 'Rules' Virgo and Gemini. They were unaware that the Planetary relationships with the Signs are based, as all Astrology is, on geometry. We call those geometric structures "The Planetary Triangles", which are shown in the following chapter.

At the time of their discovery it was believed that these newly discovered Planets, that orbit beyond the limits of the naked eye, influenced humans in the same way as those Planets which humanity has been observing for eons. As modern studies in human physiology show us, humans are not wired that way.

The body's perceptual limitations define an object's influence. The phrases 'Out of sight out of mind', and 'I only believe what I can see', demonstrate how most of humanity operates. The result of those Astrologers rearranging the Tables was a weird, sexist, ineffective variation that became widely accepted in the modern literature.

What They Changed That We've Restored

The Rulers of the Sun, Moon, Mercury and Venus are the same in the both the Traditional and Modern systems.

- ☉ The Sun Rules Dynamic ♌ Leo
- ☽ The Moon Rules Receptive ♋ Cancer
- ☿ Mercury Rules Dynamic ♊ Gemini & Receptive ♍ Virgo
- ♀ Venus Rules Receptive ♉ Taurus & Dynamic ♎ Libra

In the Traditional System
- ♂ Mars Rules Dynamic ♈ Aries & Receptive ♏ Scorpio
- ♃ Jupiter Rules Dynamic ♐ Sagittarius & Receptive ♓ Pisces
- ♄ Saturn Rules Receptive ♑ Capricorn & Dynamic ♒ Aquarius

That was as far as the human eye could consistently see!

In the Modern Rulers the Signs for Mars, Jupiter and Saturn were split apart and given to Uranus, Neptune and Pluto.

♂ Mars continued to Rule Dynamic ♈ Aries
♃ Jupiter continued to Rule Dynamic ♐ Sagittarius
♄ Saturn continued to Rule Receptive ♑ Capricorn
♅ Uranus assumed the Rulership of Dynamic ♒ Aquarius
♆ Neptune assumed the Rulership of Receptive ♓ Pisces
♇ Pluto assumed the Rulership of Receptive ♏ Scorpio

Let's start with Saturn who is related to old age and is generally the least favorite Planet. They took Saturn's Masculine Sign Aquarius, and gave it to the new guy in town, Uranus, named for the Sky God. Tellingly, even though Saturn was stuck with the Feminine Sign Capricorn as its solitary Sign, the Planet is still considered symbolic of Old Man Time? Why not Old Woman Time? Because there are six Signs that relate to Saturn and four of them are Masculine. While Saturn has a feminine side too, he is just not very in touch with it! Yet, those Astrologers chose to leave Feminine Capricorn as the sole Sign under the domain of serious, often maligned Saturn.

Next, they took the Feminine Signs away from the most adventurous Planets, Mars and Jupiter, and sent them to the denizens of the eternal night; Neptune and Pluto. Scorpio and Pisces are the quintessential expression of the powerful, mysterious nature of women, that the Astrologers chose to banish to a deep, eternally dark space.

Thanks to those changes, the Table went from an insightful Astrological tool, to an obscure artifact that students learned about but barely used. By disconnecting the Table from its geometry, those Astrologers inadvertently tilted the field towards a mystical, esoteric and psychological approach. This was a bumpy detour for what was once considered the 'Queen of the Sciences'. Fortunately, 'science' is the operative word here. Remember, these changes in the Table happened before the first space flights, the great telescopes, computers, the world wide web and modern theorems in Physics. These advances have promoted an Astrological Renaissance that has put the art back on a path that attracts and promotes human brilliance.

In the Table we use, we have returned the lost Signs of Saturn, Jupiter and Mars, but we have one more item that needs to be corrected in alignment with the geometry. In current tables, the Sun and the Moon are each assigned four Signs; one Ruling, one Exalted, one Detriment and one Fall. That's unbalanced, so based on the Planetary Triangles, we've assigned them the normal complement of Rulers and Detriments. This is not an entirely original idea. Some ancient Tables gave the Sun and Moon shared Rulership over Leo and Cancer. But, based on the geometry, we've assigned Cancer as the Sun's secondary Ruler and Sagittarius as the Moon's secondary Ruler. In the next chapter we explain this in detail.

A Primer on the Function of the Dignities in Traditional Terms
In the next chapter we update the titles, but here we are using the archaic one to help you make the transition. Each of the seven visible Bodies; Sun, Moon, Mercury, Venus, Mars, Jupiter and Saturn (collectively called the Planets) connects to six Signs.

Those six relationships are formed into two groups, or triangles. The first triplicity is; the Masculine Ruler, the Feminine Ruler and the Exalted Sign. The second triplicity is; the Masculine Detriment, the Feminine Detriment and the Fall Sign. For example, Mercury Rules Masculine Gemini and Feminine Virgo and is Exalted in Aquarius. The Detriment Signs are Masculine Sagittarius and Feminine Pisces and the Fall Sign is Leo.
The titles are unhelpfully arcane so in the next chapter we've updated them. Graphic of Mercury Table

The Planets beyond Saturn, the Asteroids and the 'Fixed Stars' affect life on Earth, but they are not the main players in our game. Symbolically, Saturn is the visible wall of our Solar village and Uranus, Neptune and Pluto travel outside that protective circle. Uranus was discovered just as the American and French Revolutions were brewing. It can represent the revolutionaries, outlaws, eccentrics and inventors. Neptune was discovered during the Spiritualist movement and the invention of the phonograph, photo film, movies and the wide-scale use of electricity.

It relates to the pervasive influence of intuition, spiritual belief, the media, movies and manufactured illusions. Pluto is a very small, complex Planet that was discovered at the dawn of the atomic age, the invention of penicillin and the computer, so it relates to issues of global power and survival; energy generation and bombs, manufactured medicines and pathogens, innovative materials and pollution, genetic manipulation and overpopulation. These three Planets all have long orbits, beyond the average age of humans, so they affect multiple generations, entire populations over extended timelines. Most of humanity today will never see these three with their own eyes, just in photos, so those Planets don't get a spot on our personal chess board.

We feel that our reasoning about the assignments of the Signs and Planets is valid, supported by the geometry, current science and our professional work in Location and Health Astrology; two very practical, results oriented areas. We simply find that the traditional assignments better reflect what we observe. Never forget that Astrology is an experiential art.

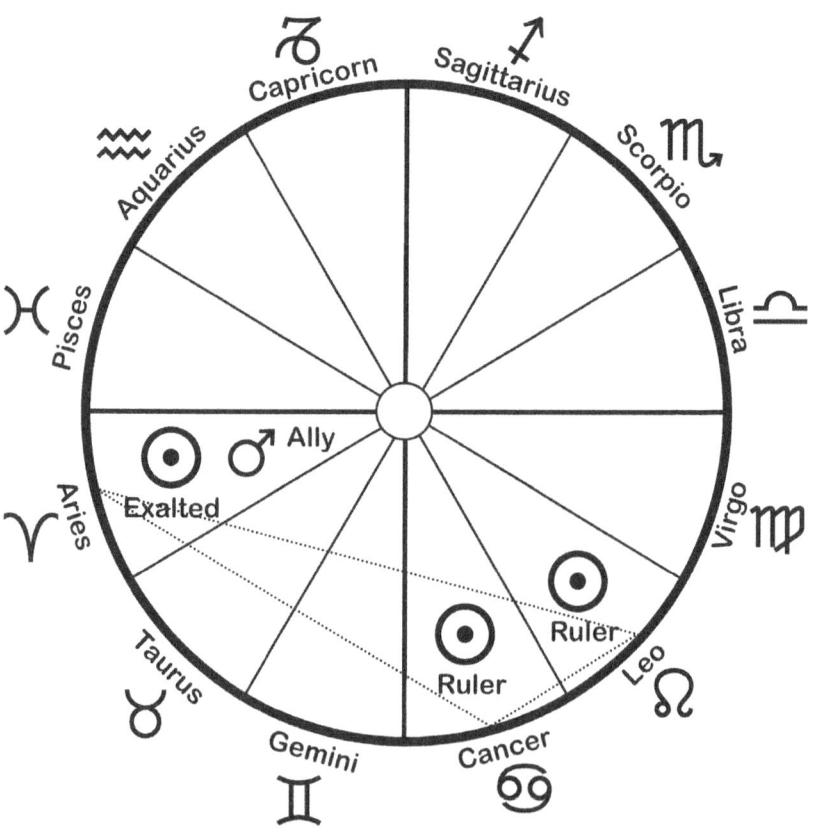

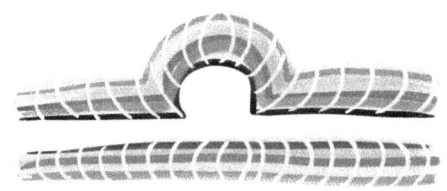

Chapter Seven: The Table of Dignities

Note: It is a common practice to call all the orbiting Celestial bodies, including the Sun and Moon the 'Planets'.

The Table of Dignities, in use since antiquity, tells us the relative strengths and unique roles of the Planets when they are in the different Signs; which are the leaders, and which are the followers in a Chart, which Planets are their colleagues, and which are their confidantes? These roles are called the Dignities. It's a wonderful system for Chart interpretation, but for many years, using it has been difficult.

That's because, after the discovery of Uranus, Neptune and Pluto, misogynistic Astrologers, ignorant of the geometry that makes the Table work, broke it! They did this by haphazardly stealing Signs from the visible Planets and giving them to the new kids on the block. It turned this logical, geometric marvel into an unworkable tool.

Through our research, we've restored the original geometry to the Table, and hopefully, begun to undo the damage caused by having this wonderful tool sidelined for so long. We'll demonstrate the Geometry at each step, to make it easier to understand and remember the Dignities.

Note: The entire system is based on Triangles.

The Dignities in Their Table

The Table of Rulers Based on the Planetary Triangles						
Celestial Body	Dynamic Ruler	Receptive Ruler	Exalted Sign	Dynamic Detriment	Receptive Detriment	Fall Sign
☉	♌	♋ v	♈	♒	♑ v	♎
☾	♐ v	♋	♉	♊ v	♑	♏
☿	♊	♍	♒	♐	♓	♌
♀	♎	♉	♓	♈	♏	♍
♂	♈	♏	♑	♎	♉	♋
♃	♐	♓	♋	♊	♍	♑
♄	♑	♒	♎	♋	♌	♈
⚳	♊	♍	♏	♐	♓	♉

Dotted Line Designates a Primary Sign & V a Vice Sign. www.SpaceAndTime.com (C) 2018 R & L De Amicis

Each Planet has a Masculine Ruling Sign and a Feminine Ruling Sign. For example, Jupiter Rules Sagittarius and Pisces. When a Planet is in a Ruling Sign, it leads the way and initiates activities related to the talents of that Planet. For example, Jupiter in Ruling Sagittarius fully expresses Jove's boundless love for travel, while in Pisces its imagination and compassion are allowed full expression. There is a third 'Ruling' Sign called the Exalted Sign.

When a Planet is in that Sign it also initiates activities related to that Planet. The difference is, the Exalted Sign has a side-deal with another Planet. We know which Planet it's allied with because the Sign of the Exaltation is also the 'Ruling Sign' of another Planet. So, when a Planet is in the Exalted Sign, while carrying out the actions of the first Planet, it is also operating in accord with that second Planet, no matter where it is in the Chart. For example, Jupiter is Exalted in Cancer, the Ruling Sign of the Moon, so in that Sign Jupiter has a nurturing, reflective quality in its expression. The Moon, no matter what Sign it's occupying, is made more effective by that alliance.

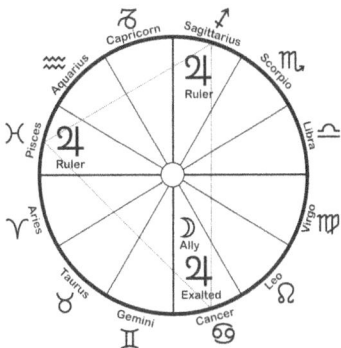

The Jupiter Ruling Triplicity and the Allied Planet

Here is another example: Saturn's Ruling Signs are Capricorn and Aquarius, and in those Signs the Saturnian drive for long-term accomplishment is fully expressed. Saturn is Exalted in Libra, showing the desire to accomplish those activities in partnership with others, which is often a key to success. Libra is a Ruling Sign of Venus, so Saturn in Libra carries out the ambitious Saturnian agenda, while being aligned with Venusian ethics; fairness, co-operation, and commitment. In the Natal Chart, Saturn in Libra is ambitious, but its actions are complimentary to that of Venus, irrespective of the Sign Venus is occupying, which is fortunate for Venus, because Saturn in Libra is a good ally.

The Saturn Ruling Triplicity and the Allied Planet

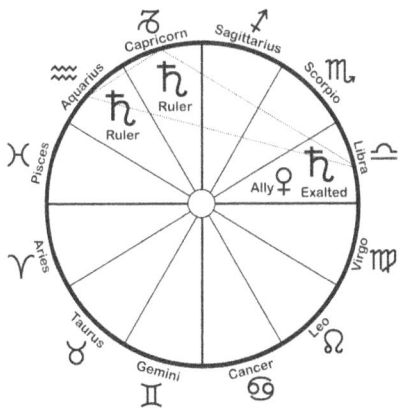

The Detriments

The two Signs opposite the Rulers are called the Detriments. When the Planet is in those Signs, it is a follower. Instead of initiating, it reacts to events related to that Planet. The Sign opposite the Exalted Sign is called the Fall Sign. It is also reactive to the activities of the first Planet, but it has an affinity with the Planet for which that is a Ruling Sign.

The Mercury Ruling & Detriment Triplicities

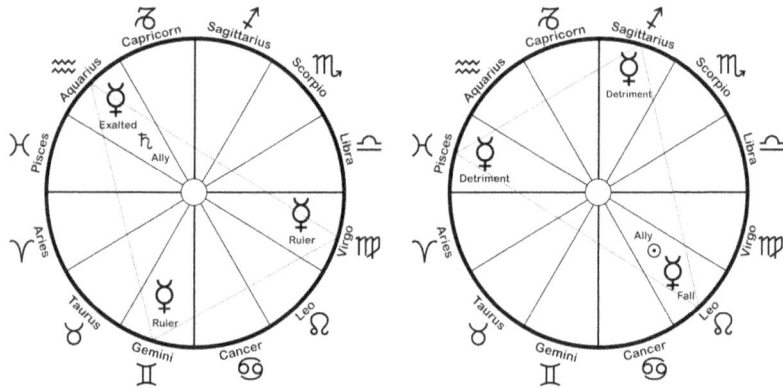

For example, Mercury's Ruling Signs are Masculine Gemini and Feminine Virgo. The Exalted Sign is Aquarius. The opposite Signs, Sagittarius and Pisces are Mercury's Detriment Signs and the Fall Sign is Leo. When Mercury is in a Ruling Sign in a Natal Chart, that person is confident initiating communications, exploring, interacting and exchanging ideas. In a Detriment Sign, the person tends to depend on others to initiate the contact and choose the subject, at which point they become very effective, because they're a natural supporter in the Mercurial equation, comfortable navigating an area that someone else has mapped.

Mercury in the Exalted Sign Aquarius is connected to Saturn, and that position's ability to widely network supports both Mercury and Saturn's social, ambitious goals. In comparison, the opposite Fall Sign, Leo, is connected to the Sun, and Mercury in

Leo's ability to produce supportive self-talk serves both Mercury and the Sun's desires for engagement and personal enhancement.

The Ruling and Exalted Signs are happiest out in the open, while the Detriment and Fall Signs are most comfortable behind the scenes. It may be helpful to imagine the Planet as an actor in a Summer Stock theater group, where each troupe member does different tasks, depending on the play. In three of the Signs, the Rulers and Exaltation, the Planet plays a character on stage. In the three opposite Signs, the Detriments and Fall, the Planets work backstage, supporting the production.

On a psychological level, we define the Ruler, or Leader as an Extrovert, because the place where its actions matter to it are External. The relationship between the Ruling Signs and the Exalted is friendly, or collegial, so we call the Exalted Sign the 'Colleague'. We define the Detriment, or Follower as an Introvert because the place where its actions matter to it are Internal. The relationship between the Detriments and the Fall Sign is also friendly but concealed, so we call it the 'Confidante'. If the two Rulers are the Male and Female lead on the stage, the Exalted Sign is the supporting actor. The two Detriments are behind the scenes running the lights and the sound, and the Fall Sign is the makeup artist.

How the Table of Dignities Connect the Planets to the Signs

Imagine each Planet as a parent, the Ruling Signs are the twin son and daughter, who are equal in power and talent, but different in expression. The Exalted Sign is the twin's best friend and later in life, when they go out to make their mark on the world, their Colleague. Imagine the Detriment Signs as the same Planet's other twin son and daughter. Unlike the Ruling siblings, these Twins stayed at home and worked on the family farm or business. From years of hard work, they're a sturdy pair and a great help, but not as polished or outgoing as their 'city siblings'.

These Twins have a childhood friend and confidante, who knows all their secrets, and now works besides them, called the Fall Sign.

When a sole Planet in a Natal Chart is in a Ruling Sign, it takes the lead in the external, visible agenda. Equally a sole Detriment can take the lead of the internal, invisible agenda. For example, if Venus in Taurus is the Chart's sole Ruling Sign, that person's interests in food, gardening, interior design, finance and romance will dominate. When a sole Planet is Exalted or in Fall, it gives up some command, for leverage.

When several Planets are in Ruling positions, that's like several talented athletes competing on the same team, if they can all find opportunities to express themselves, then success is assured. However, multiple Rulers can so monopolize the outer life that the personal life suffers for lack of attention. When the Detriment positions dominate, the focus on personal growth, family issues, wellbeing and health may deny the person outer success.

The Dignities in Their Table

The Table of Rulers Based on the Planetary Triangles						
Celestial Body	Dynamic Ruler	Receptive Ruler	Exalted Sign	Dynamic Detriment	Receptive Detriment	Fall Sign
☉	Leo	Cancer (v)	Aries	Aquarius	Capricorn (v)	Libra
☽	Sagittarius (v)	Cancer	Taurus	Gemini (v)	Capricorn	Scorpio
☿	Gemini	Virgo	Aquarius	Sagittarius	Pisces	Leo
♀	Libra	Taurus	Pisces	Aries	Scorpio	Virgo
♂	Aries	Scorpio	Capricorn	Libra	Taurus	Cancer
♃	Sagittarius	Pisces	Cancer	Gemini	Virgo	Capricorn
♄	Capricorn	Aquarius	Libra	Cancer	Leo	Aries
♇	Gemini	Virgo	Scorpio	Sagittarius	Pisces	Taurus

Dotted Line Designates a Primary Sign & V a Vice Sign. www.SpaceAndTime.com (C) 2018 R & L De Amicis

***The Ruling and Detriment positions
each feed a different part of our souls.***

Planets possessing no Dignity in a Chart are 'Wild Cards', dependent upon the power of positioning; Aspects and their proximity to an Angle to determine their effectiveness. While the Dignities are the Planetary genetics, Aspects and Angles carry the power of strategic positioning. It's rare that a Chart has no Planets in Dignity, but in that case the dominant Planet is determined by its position.

Interesting Conjunctions

What happens when you have a Planet in its Ruling Sign, Conjunct a Planet in its Detriment Sign? It's like a good marriage; the two players gain from each other's viewpoint and connections! The Ruling Sign accesses the Detriment's depth, while the Detriment accesses the Ruling Signs expressive outlets. They make each other better!

For example, if Venus in Virgo is Conjunct Mercury in Virgo, Venus now has a pathway to love and relationships through Mercury's silver tongue. While Mercury gains the Venusian understanding of relationships that its quick wit often misses. Here's another example. When Mars in its Ruling Sign Aries, is Conjunct Venus in its Detriment Sign Aries, that single-minded Martial approach receives an infusion of Venusian gracefulness, that makes that Martian boldness more attractive. In relationships, that self-centered approach to relationships can be validated by the bravery that Mars brings to the game of love. *"A faint heart never won a fair lady".*

The Planetary Positions and Relationships

The Dignities are listed in this order:
1) Masculine Ruling 2) Feminine Ruling 3) Exalted Sign
4) Masculine Detriment 5) Feminine Detriment 6) Fall Sign

The ☉ Sun has domain over the Ruling Twins: Masculine ♌ Leo & Feminine ♋ Cancer. The Exalted Sign is Masculine ♈ Aries (related to Mars). The Detriment Twins are: Masculine ♒ Aquarius & Feminine ♑ Capricorn. The Fall Sign is Masculine ♎ Libra (related to Venus)

The ☽ Moon has domain over the Ruling Twins: Feminine ♋ Cancer & Masculine ♐ Sagittarius. The Exalted Sign is Feminine ♉ Taurus (related to Venus). The Detriment Twins are: Feminine ♑ Capricorn & Masculine ♊ Gemini. The Fall Sign is Feminine ♏ Scorpio (related to Mars)

☿ Mercury has domain over the Ruling Twins: Masculine ♊ Gemini & Feminine ♍ Virgo. The Exalted Sign is Masculine ♒ Aquarius (related to Saturn). The Detriment Twins are: Masculine ♐ Sagittarius & Feminine ♓ Pisces. The Fall Sign is Masculine ♌ Leo (related to the Sun)

♀ Venus has domain over the Ruling Twins: Masculine ♎ Libra & Feminine ♉ Taurus. The Exalted Sign is Feminine Pisces ♓ (related to Jupiter). The Detriment Twins are: Masculine ♈ Aries & Feminine ♏ Scorpio. The Fall Sign is Feminine ♍ Virgo (related to Mercury)

♂ Mars has domain over the Ruling Twins: Masculine ♈ Aries & Feminine ♏ Scorpio. The Exalted Sign is Feminine ♑ Capricorn (related to Saturn). The Detriment Twins are: Masculine ♎ Libra & Feminine ♉ Taurus. The Fall Sign is Feminine ♋ Cancer (related to the Moon)

♃ Jupiter has domain over the Ruling Twins: Masculine ♐ Sagittarius & Feminine ♓ Pisces. The Exalted Sign is Feminine ♋ Cancer (related to the Moon). The Detriment Twins are: Masculine ♊ Gemini & Feminine ♍ Virgo. The Fall Sign is Feminine ♑ Capricorn (related to Saturn)

♄ Saturn has domain over the Ruling Twins: Masculine ♒ Aquarius & Feminine ♑ Capricorn. The Exalted Sign is Masculine ♎ Libra (related to Venus). The Detriment Twins are: Masculine ♌ Leo & Feminine ♋ Cancer. The Fall Sign is Masculine ♈ Aries (related to Mars)

The Dignities in People's Charts

Famous people and movie stars often have multiple Planets in Ruling and Detriment positions, making them easily recognizable no matter what role they play thanks to the Ruling Signs, and able to plumb their depths due to the Detriment Signs.

The actress Natalie Wood had every Planet in either a Ruling or Detriment position, so she was able to reach great depths in her performances and yet, audiences could easily identify with her. Curiously many successful, but less recognizable actors have no Dignified Planets. This flexibility allows them to disappear seamlessly into various roles and not become typecast.

The Ruling qualities are made available to the world, while the Detriment qualities are kept for personal use. Abraham Lincoln had every major Planet in a Detriment position, indicating great depth, except Jupiter in the Feminine Ruling Sign of Pisces. In some ways he was more than his countryman's President, he was their Shaman. His intense inner life and focus was expressed externally through a narrow Jovian (Jupiter) outlet, which by itself, has a deep capacity for enduring suffering for a spiritual cause.

Oprah Winfrey has a powerful mix, with her ego denying Detriment Sun in Masculine Aquarius, a super-charged Mars in Ruling Feminine Scorpio and a brilliant Masculine Exalted Mercury in Aquarius, making her perfect for both the media and as a manager of a large organization. Her powerful Sagittarius Moon, strategically placed in the fourth House opposite Jupiter in

Detriment Gemini, brings great humanity and generosity to her career. Taken together, it makes her easy to recognize and relate to, while communicating her willingness to focus on the group's benefits rather than her own.

In a Chart, the Ruling and Detriment positions are both prominent in their own arenas. The Exalted and Fall Signs show us where, among the Planets, they find allies. This network of compacts reflects the web of social relationships that humans live within every day. When Planets are connected by significant positions, it shows that the person has an open channel between these qualities.

For example, Mercury's Exalted Sign is Aquarius, showing a connection to Saturn. This describes an open phone line between the young and old parts of the personality, rather like the natural alliance that exists between grandchildren and grandparents.

When we move beyond a shallow, good or bad judgement of the Ruling and Detriment positions, to an understanding of the interactive nuances, it can provide tremendous insights because, just like anyone who has ever watched Judge Judy knows, relationships are rarely all good or bad, but they are often complicated.

For sake of completion and ease of reference, the following two pages show the rest of the Planetary Triplicities

The Table of Dignities 77

The Moon Triplicities

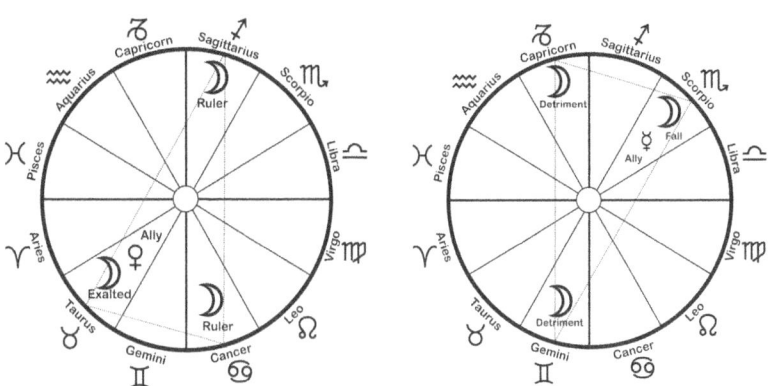

The Sun Triplicities

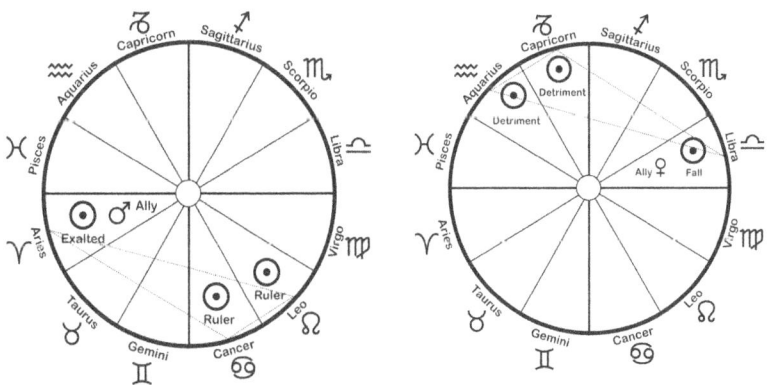

Venus Triplicities

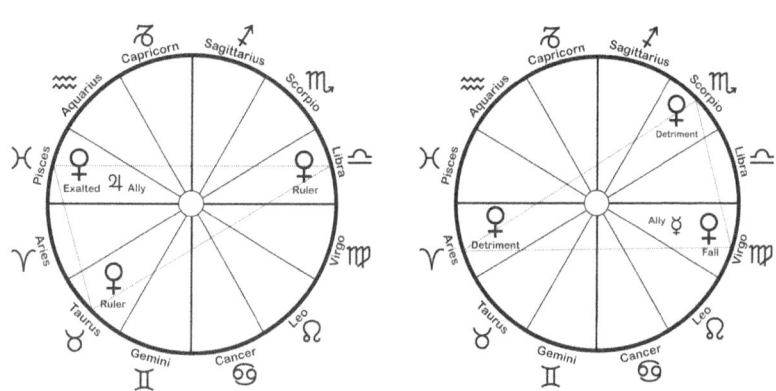

Mars Triplicities

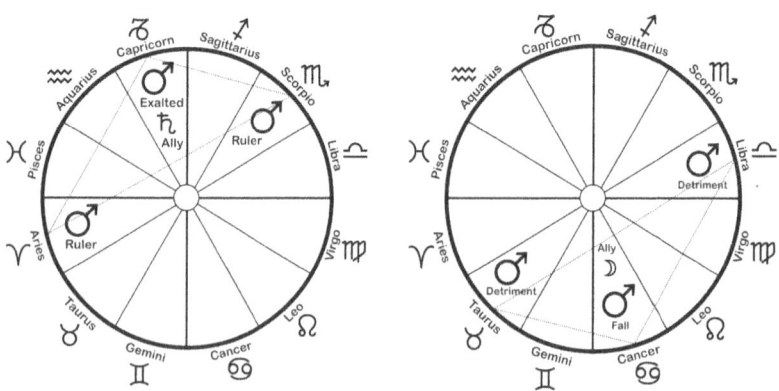

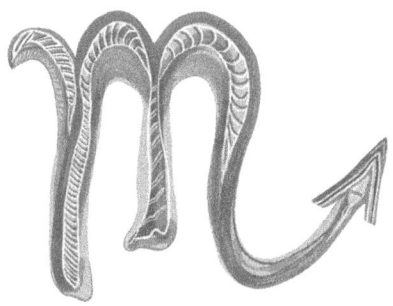

Chapter Eight: The Aspects, Transits & You

Aspects are the Angles, measured in degrees, between the Celestial Bodies. Planets can also form Aspects to the primary angles; Ascendant, Descendant, Midheaven and IC. The network of Aspects and Rulerships is the Chart's wiring diagram. It shows how the players either support, challenge or ignore each other. It's like understanding a family or team, you can know the individuals, but only when you know the relationships do you understand how they work and play together, for better or worse. The Rulerships in the Table of Dignities describe the underlying nature of those relationships.

The Traditional Aspects measured in Longitude (East to West) are the Conjunction (0 to 7 Degrees), the Sextile (60 Degrees), the Square (90 Degrees), the Trine (120 Degrees) and the Opposition (180 Degrees).

The Esoteric Aspects are The Quintile (72 Degrees) and The Quincunx (150 Degrees).
The Aspects measured in Latitude (North to South) are the Parallel and the Contra Parallel.

You have seen these Aspects your whole life, while watching the Phases of the Moon. So to demonstrate these Aspects in action we are using the Moon's Phases, which are the various distances between the Sun to the Moon. They exist between every Planet.

Conjunction

The Conjunction is the New Moon. The Sun and Moon are together in the sky, so the nights are Moonless, the darkes of the month and the energy levels are at a low ebb. It is both the end of a cycle and the beginning of another. The two Lights are unified in their message, like a couple coming to a decision and acting together. When the Moon and Sun are both aligned east to west and north to south (Parallel), the Moon passes in front of the Sun in a Solar Eclipse, signifying that the Emotional needs are eclipsing the Spiritual agenda.

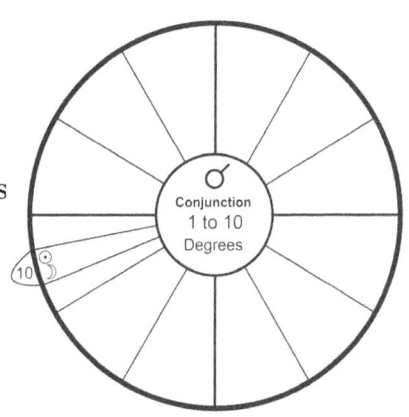

Sextile

The Sextile (60 degrees) is the Crescent Moon following the New Moon, creating an easy, supportive connection, like cousins shopping together.

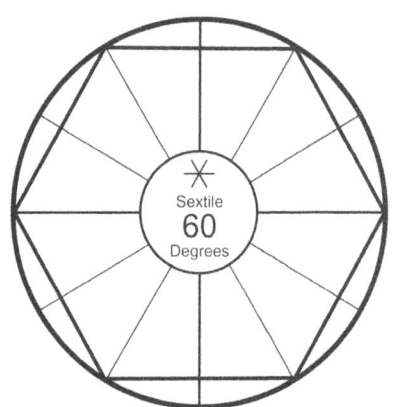

Square

The Square (90 degrees) is the Half Moon, also called the quarter Moon, the Sun and Moon are at right angles, like encountering a car an intersection, you work together to determine who is going first.

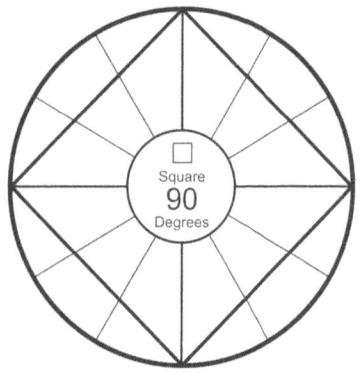

Trine

The Trine (120 degrees) is the Gibbous Moon, or three-quarter Moon. The two are in a harmonious, strongly supportive connection, like siblings planning an event together for their parent.

Opposition

The Opposition (180 degrees) is the Full Moon. When the Sun and Moon are opposite each other, like two people sitting across from each other negotiating, each will need to loosen their grasp on their own position in order to find common ground. But, that

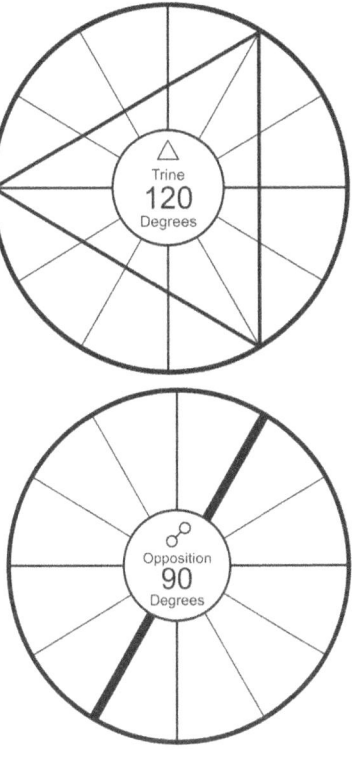

sacrifice comes with a reward, greater fulfillment; the Sun's light is fully reflected and the Moon is brightly shining regent of the night. It is a time when spiritual and emotional messages, although opposite, are fully expressed. When the Sun and Moon are also aligned north to south the Earth is exactly between the and that is a Lunar Eclipse. The symbolizes the material matters are overshadowing the emotional needs.

After the Full Moon Opposition, the series of Aspects happens in reverse; Trine, Square, Sextile and finally the Conjunction at the next New Moon. For practical reasons, it is good to note the Waning Trine and Sextile following the Full Moon, when the Sun and Moon have made their positions clear. Because everything has been brought into the open and now, they are at a harmonious position, a Trine is a good time to aggressively move projects along and a Sextile is perfect for wrapping it up.

These same Aspects happen between all the Planets and they create the varying subtle levels of tension and ease that we experience on Earth.

Transits

One of the ways Astrology helps us in our daily life is by recognizing how the traveling (Transiting) Planets affect us through these Aspects. While the Birth (Natal) Chart represents that unique moment of incarnation, the Celestial Bodies don't stop in their orbits. Their Transits through the Signs shape our experience in predictable ways. We use that knowledge to Forecast future conditions, by looking at what happened last time those Transits formed.

The repeating pattern doesn't give us the whole picture, because other Bodies are influencing the situation, but it will still provide valuable information. The more Planets you can bring into the equation the better the predictions. Forecasting is a bit like horse racing; you research the past performance, consider the current situation and then make your bet.

Each Transiting Celestial Body's effect is unique. Having Venus in Libra visit is very different from Saturn in Libra dropping by for a chat. The first is your girlfriend arriving with a bottle of wine, while the second is grandma at your door for tea, with a box of your baby pictures. The Aspect between any Transiting and Natal body creates an influential pressure, the angle determines the type of leverage at work.

How Do the Players Shape the Aspect?

The prominence of the Celestial Body making the Aspect matters, because the Lights and Planets exist in a hierarchy and their strength or vulnerability vary, as shown in the Table of Dignities. It is like different characters on a stage delivering lines; their role, script and costume colors the impression they make. While a prominent character is hard to ignore, a bit player may come and go on stage with barely a notice. So, Saturn, with that serious voice, passing over your Sun will get your attention for an extended period, but a quick Opposition of Mercury over your Natal Midheaven will register as a brief but entertaining chirp.

Here is a snapshot of how some of the players act on stage. Jupiter (the bold entrepreneur) expands issues while Saturn (the respected elder) restricts them. When Saturn Conjuncts your Natal Jupiter, it clamps down on Jove's enthusiasm. The Ruling Signs of Venus (the artistic youth), Taurus and Libra, are opposite those of Mars, (the energetic youth) Aries and Scorpio. While a Transiting Mars Conjunction empowers you to action, a Transiting Venus Conjunction harmonizes and indulges your desire for relaxation.

Because Saturn is Exalted (honored) in Libra (Venus's Ruling Sign), and Mercury is Exalted in Aquarius (Saturn's Ruling Sign), Mercury and Venus enjoy a special relationship with Saturn (the respected elder), like grandchildren loving their indulgent grandparents. A visit from the Grandparents delights the grandchildren, although it may drive the Dad and Mom (Sun and Moon) a little crazy. That is because Saturn is connected to the parents through the Introvert-Detriment relationships, so Saturn Aspects to the Sun and Moon instill a sense of vulnerability.

These connections defined by the Dignities shows how they interact, based on their power and position. It's complicated, which is why having a good understanding of the Dignities is like going to the theater and be handed the playbill, which explains the backstory for the characters in a play. The Transiting Aspects people notice most are to the Sun, Moon and Natal Ascendant. After that, Transits involving quickly moving Mercury, Venus or Mars are felt most personally. The Transits involving slower moving Jupiter and Saturn, as well as those to the Natal Midheaven, are experienced externally, because they paint with a broader brush and their arena is the outer world.

Transits involving Uranus, Neptune and Pluto, whose motions are very slow, often feel impersonal, as if the tide is rising and the perspective from the boat deck is gradually changing for everyone aboard. Those outer Planet Transits are a very different experience from, 'Bam! Wake Up, Mars is Here!'

Understanding How the Aspects Function

We previously discussed the three ways that Signs are determined; Polarity, Element and Quality. It is the various connections between these that form the five traditional Aspects. An Aspect makes a connection that is either supportive or challenging, but that doesn't necessarily mean beneficial or detrimental. There is a tendency to simplify the definitions, saying that Sextiles and Trines being supportive are good, while Squares and Oppositions are challenging and bad. Conjunctions can be either good or bad, depending on the players. For example, Venus Conjunct Mercury in Gemini brings wit, charm and flexibility. On the other hand, Saturn Conjunct Mars in Taurus will create an indestructible stubborn streak. Defining something as good or bad also depends on the situation and the talents needed, so look at the Planets involved.

In a general sense it's true that the Supportive Aspects are easy and don't take a lot of effort. The Challenging Aspects are harder, taking grit and effort to make them work properly. But it depends on the bodies making the connection and the results it yields. It's nice when things are easy, and it can be unpleasant when things get rough, but often your best allies are those people that challenge you to be better.

For example, Gemini and Virgo Sun Signs frequently work in the same industries. They are both Ruled by Mercury and they form a Square, but the operative word here is 'work', that is the place where the Square shines! The same thing happens with Sagittarius and Pisces Sun Signs, both are Ruled by Jupiter and form a Square. These two are often found in both entrepreneurial and non-profit organizations, working side by side. The shared Planetary Rulership draws them to the same fields while the Square recognizes that there will be challenges that need to be overcome.

Sometimes your worst allies are those that support your bad habits. It depends on what the Conjunction, Sextile and Trine support. Another way to understand the difference is this; supportive Aspects create stability while challenging Aspects create change.

A Brief Survey of The Five Traditional Aspects

1) The Conjunction connects Planets within a Sign (0 to 5 or 10 Degrees) aligning their actions. 2) The supportive Sextile connects the closest Signs of the same Polarity (60 Degrees) that provide a helping hand when needed. 3) The challenging Square connects adjacent Signs of the same Quality (90 Degrees) stimulating action and competition. 4) The supportive Trine connects Signs of the same Polarity and Element (120 Degrees) that help each other continually. 5) The challenging Opposition connects Signs of the same Polarity and Quality (180 Degrees) offering the opposing point of view.

The T Square and Cross

When three Planets are in Signs of the same Quality, connected through two Squares and an Opposition, it is called a T-Square and it shows a focused method for accomplishment. For example, a Cardinal T Square shows a propensity for initiating projects and getting things done. When there is also a Planet in the fourth Sign that is called Grand Cross and it shows a person compelled to follow a certain path, because they are always attempting to balance opposing demands and it forces them to the middle way. This may be the result of them being born into a situation where their familial tradition and responsibilities circumscribe their aspirations.

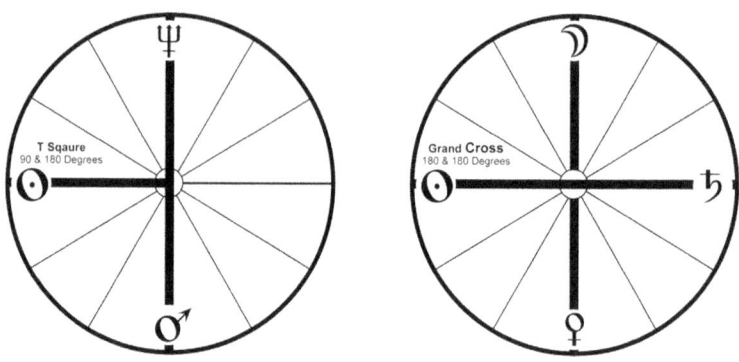

The Grand Trine

When Planets are connected by Trines between all three Signs of an Element that is called a Grand Trine and it shows a special aptitude for that Elemental talent. A person with a Grand Fire Trine will demonstrate a high level of creativity, an interest in people and social change. A Grand Trine in Earth will show a talent in finance, culinary arts and business. The Grand Air Sign expresses through a talent in communications, social organizations and cooperative ventures.

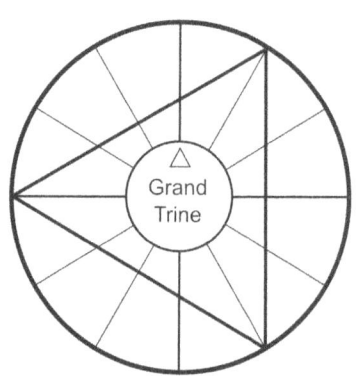

The Quintile and Quincunx

There are numerous minor Aspects that are used by Astrologers. But among those are some powerful Esoteric Aspects that carry very specific messages. The highly creative Quintile (72 Degrees) accesses the deeper areas of human potential. The trans-dimensional Quincunx (150 Degrees) accesses Angelic communication pathways.

These two Aspects do not make their connections through the Polarities, Qualities or Elements. Their magic comes from other avenues.

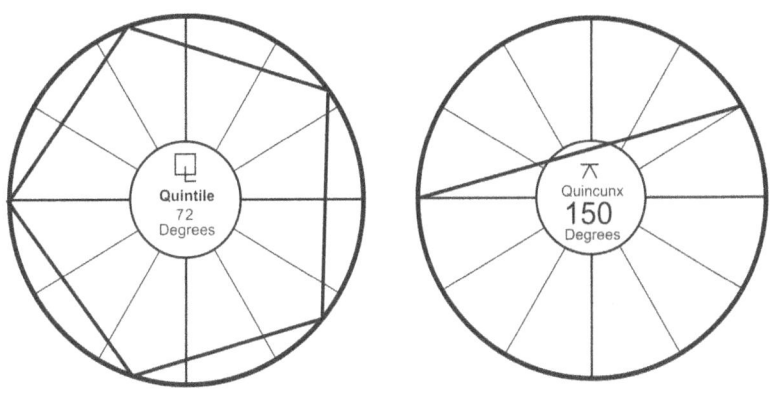

The 'Orb of Influence'

When are two Celestial bodies solidly connected by an Aspect? When they are within the 'Orb of Influence'. That traditionally means up to 10 degrees of the exact angle. Example: The Sun at 1 degree Aries and Mercury at 1 degree Aries are exactly Conjunct (called Partile), but as quick Mercury moves away that connection becomes weaker.

At a 5-degree separation it is still very active, but by 10-degrees the connection become nebulous and by 11 degrees even the most generous Astrologer will consider it disconnected. In familial terms, if the exact Aspect is the connection between siblings, a 5 degrees separation connects first cousins, and a ten degrees separation relates to second cousins. It's not as strong, but hey, they're still family!

About Aspects

As you personally encounter Transiting Aspects through time, you develop a library of experiences that inform your understanding of the Celestial Bodies and yourself. You will find that

Transits made by the Sun and Moon are applied with a broad stroke, while the Planets are specific in their message. Conjunctions give you the clearest insight into the nature of the Celestial Body because the experience is intimate. When you encounter an Aspect, notice what activities come easily, giving you pleasure and satisfaction, and which challenge you and bring you grief.

Notice how your body feels, flexible or stiff, drained or energized. Your conscious awareness and acknowledgment of these influences will expand your knowledge, and help you understand your emotions, reactions and experiences. This process is an important tool for your personal growth and over time, you will expand your knowledge and enjoyment of the 'Starry Arts'. Facilitating that process is the reason that the Planetary Calendar exists.

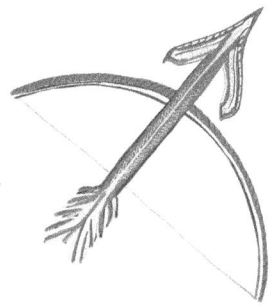

Chapter Nine: Calendars, Seasons & Forecasts

All calendars are based on Planetary motions. Traditionally, the main differences between them are how many celestial bodies they are based on and which astronomical alignments each culture considers significant. Of course, sometimes astronomical tradition is forgotten, as in the West, where we celebrate the first day of the year on January First. That date has no connection to any significant, repeating Planetary alignment.

That is because our popular calendar is overdue to be reset to a seasonally significant start date, something that needs to be done with almost all calendars periodically. In ancient China, when the Royal Astrologers considered the current calendar too far out of sync with the seasons, they would use the ascension of a new Dynasty to reset the date.

Our current calendar was last reset twenty centuries ago by Julius Caesar, with the help of Alexandrian Astrologers. They replaced the Roman Lunar calendar, with its movable days, with the Solar Julian calendar in 45 BCE. They started it on the day of a sunrise Eclipse in Rome; very dramatic and sure to get everyone's attention! While its year was accurately based on the movement of the Sun related to the equinoxes, it was not perfect.

So, in 1582 the current Gregorian calendar, an improvement on the Julian, was introduced. It is also not perfect, although it comes closer to solving the problem of the year being about five hours, forty-eight minutes and forty-five seconds longer than 365 days. The mechanism for making the calendar come out right is the Leap Day, but even this imperfect solution still allows the calendar to gradually get out of sync with the equinoxes.

Our modern arrangement requires society to maintain two calendars; the Gregorian 'day counter', that starts on January first, and a seasonal calendar that defines the year through the Equinoxes (the first days of Spring and Fall), Solstices (the first days of Summer and Winter) and the Phases of the Moon. For living on Earth, knowing these seasonal and Lunar markers is more essential to our health and wellbeing. Yet, they are recorded inside the Gregorian calendar and we've become accustomed to connecting April to Spring and December to Winter.

The importance of these Celestially timed markers is obvious. Society celebrates the beginning of each of the four seasons; the Spring festivals are April Fools and Easter, the Summer festivals are Memorial Day and July Fourth, the Autumn festivals are Labor Day and Octoberfest and the Winter festivals are Hanukkah and Christmas.

Both the Autumn and Winter festivals are heavy on the alcohol, to encourage baby making to yield twins in Gemini (June) and dutiful children in Virgo (September). Those are the two Mercurial, or 'kid' Signs and births in those months are considered especially helpful in agricultural communities. In comparison, the January First 'day counter' calendar gets one festival, New Year's Eve, a night out and a boon to Champagne and confetti makers everywhere.

We depend on the seasonal calendar to time our year, manage our gardens, choose our clothing, set our heating and cooling regimens and plan our events. In the Roman Empire the year began on the first day of Spring, for us March 20th. April Fool's Day is a remnant of that festival. The Chinese Empire started their year with the Springtime festival, which we call the Chinese New Year (CNY). It is celebrated at the New Moon in Aquarius, which can be any day between January 19th and February 18th. That variability is where the concept of an early or late Spring comes from, that China celebrates with Dragons and America celebrates with Groundhogs.

Chinese Astrology is Earth centered and the New Moon in Aquarius is when the Sunlight is the weakest and the energy of the Earth is most withdrawn. It is after this Lunation that the seeds begin stirring in the dark earth.

In Western cultures, our Springtime festival is aligned with the first degree of Aries, March 19th, which can be as soon as thirty days, or long as sixty days after the Aquarius New Moon. In the temperate latitudes, Aries is when the red sprouts begin to pop out of the ground.

Why does Asia celebrate the Aquarius New Moon while the West celebrates the Vernal equinox? Most festivals are founded on agriculture and the two cultures celebrate different dominant crops. The warmer Asian culture is based on rice, grown in water, where a great deal happens beneath the translucent surface. In the West, the dominant grains are grown on dry land in colder climates. The sprouts appear later in the year after the snow has melted!

About the Seasons

What do these turning points in the year; Spring, Summer, Autumn and Winter, mean to us? It is about how the transit of the Sun through the sky changes our experience! The longest night and the longest day denote the first day of Winter and the first day of Summer. Spring and Autumn are the midpoints between those times, when day and night are equally long. Spring is followed three months later with the longest day, while Autumn is followed three months later by the longest night.

The concept of a Month is based on the motion of the Moon. The year's cycle of New and Full Moons is deeply tied to the growing cycle of plants and animals. That is why almanacs traditionally have included the best time to plant, harvest, fertilize and rest. The most complete almanac of this sort is the one created for Biodynamic farmers, which is an Astrologically based agricultural system. Most people go their whole lives without seriously considering how much the shifting seasonal light shapes our experience.

How Forecasting is Done

When Astrologers write forecasts, they look at turning points and changes; the Charts for the first day of the Seasons, the New, Quarter and Full Moons and especially the Solar and Lunar Eclipses. They look at the movements of the Planets into new Signs, their changes in direction as in their Retrograde motion, when they appear to move backwards from our point of view. In the story book of the year, these turning points are the chapter titles that describe the evolving themes. That talent for capturing a narrative and immersing one's self in that symbolic story is why Astrology is an art. It requires moving easily between the logical and creative parts of the brain.

There are many opinions about which turning points are the most significant, but the anchor we use for our yearly Forecasts is the Chinese New Year Chart (New Moon in Aquarius), which we abbreviate as CNY. It is the world's most widely celebrated Planetary alignment festival and we consider it the 'Seed Chart' out of which the future year sprouts.

As any good gardener will tell you, location matters, so we calculate Charts for cities all over the world, because each has its own experience and expression of that Chart. In the most obvious examples, where there are significant Planets overhead, we anticipate their focused energy in the coming year.

With that as our starting point, we use the Lunations, Eclipses and Planetary Ingresses to create the monthly Forecasts that appear in the Planetary Calendar. It involves a great deal of discussion and they are assembled step by step, like verses in a song.

The key to effective forecasting is to remove the filters of our own charts, as much as possible, so that the picture we paint is true to the time and easily understandable by all. We hope you enjoy this peek behind the scenes and that you find the Calendar and the Forecasts illuminating.

The Signs of the Zodiac

Birth Date: **Birth Sign:** **Element:** **Quality:** **Ruling Planet**

March 21 to April 19.....Aries ♈.......Fire.......Cardinal...........Mars ♂

April 20 to May 20......Taurus ♉.......Earth......Fixed............Venus ♀

May 21 to June 20......Gemini ♊........Air........Mutable.....Mercury ☿

June 21 to July 22.......Cancer ♋.......Water.....Cardinal........Moon ☽

July 23 to Aug 22............Leo ♌..........Fire.......Fixed................Sun ☉

Aug 23 to Sept 22..........Virgo ♍........Earth.....Mutable.....Mercury ☿

Sept 23 to Oct 22..........Libra ♎.........Air........Cardinal........Venus ♀

Oct 23 to Nov 21..........Scorpio ♏.....Water.....Fixed........Tr. Mars ♂

                                                             Modern Ruler Pluto ♇

Nov 22 to Dec 21.......Sagittarius ♐.....Fire......Mutable......Jupiter ♃

Dec 22 to Jan 19.........Capricorn ♑.....Earth....Cardinal.......Saturn ♄

Jan 20 to Feb 18..........Aquarius ♒......Air........Fixed......Tr. Saturn ♄

                                                         Modern Ruler Uranus ♅

Feb 19 to March 20........Pisces ♓.....Water.......Mutable.Tr. Jupiter ♃

                                                    Modern Ruler Neptune ♆

Tr: Traditional Ruler, related to the Table of Essential Dignities that determine relative planetary strength in a chart.
Modern Ruler, suggesting an affinity between the sign and the planet first postulated in the mid-1800's.

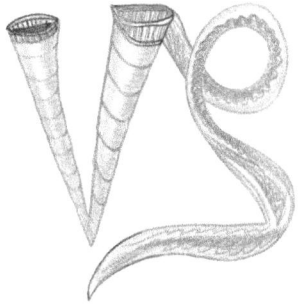

Chapter Ten: Sun Sign Spaces

Most people know their Astrological Sign, which they think of as a symbol of personality. But it equally represents the compass point on the horizon, where the Sun rises on a that specific day. That Rising point's incremental movement is how we measure time. So, think of the Signs as relating to both Space and Time.

The Sun Sign Astrology you read in the newspaper is a simplified form of a complex system. Astrology is all about the numbers and the advent of computers has been a boon for the profession. The ability to statistically analyze and tabulate charts, for studies related to health, careers and political preferences, would have been much harder without that technology.

Considering the importance of the Sun in our lives, we would expect Sol to appear as a significant indicator in multiple studies. But surprisingly, while numerous Planets are statistically significant in certain angular positions, the Sun is not! Until now, finding how the Sun makes itself known in our lives has evaded researchers.

In our experience during two plus decades of environmental consulting, the Sign of the Sun is a central indicator about the size of the Spaces where people feel comfortable and productive. It also offers clues about the types of objects they surround themselves with. We say, "As above so below", so shouldn't the Space people like reflect their Sun's preferred domain? Your Chart, your personal Solar System, with its four intimate Celestials; the Sun, Moon, Mercury and Venus, offer the best insights about Spatial preferences. The rest of the community travels outside the Earth's orbit. But these four bodies relate to family, speech, food and siblings, those shapers of our environmental habits.

We have numbered the Signs because as the numbers rise, the preference for types of surroundings expand. However, it is not exactly incremental, because the Fire and Air Signs generally like larger Spaces than the Earth and Water Signs. In comparing them, it is helpful to compare between Signs of the same Element. For example, all three Fire Signs like, brighter, high energy Spaces. But the higher the number, the larger Space they prefer, in part because they become increasingly social.

So, Aries likes a more personal Space, royal Leo likes one they can share with their subjects, and Sagittarius likes the biggest Space, outdoors is best, preferably playing a sport, which is why it is a prominent Sign among athletes.

The Signs are sequential from one to twelve: #1 Aries, #2 Taurus, #3 Gemini, #4 Cancer, #5 Leo, #6 Virgo, #7 Libra, #8 Scorpio, #9 Sagittarius, #10 Capricorn, #11 Aquarius, #12 Pisces.

They describe the stages of life from birth through growth to maturity and ultimately universality. This is the philosophical journey from "It's all about me" to "I am but a speck…" If #1 Aries is the acorn, then #10 Capricorn is the giant redwood tree. One of the obvious differences between the two is their size.

As the numbers of the Sun Signs goes up, the size of the Spaces people like gets bigger and more open

For example, we find that people with a #2 Taurus Sun tend to like cozy Spaces, muted colors and lighting. In comparison, the #11 Aquarius Sun inclines people to seek out large windows and bright Spaces. A #3 Gemini Sun likes human sized Spaces, their playful, reflective personalities also like having mirrors in their surroundings. It's not vanity that draws them to mirrors, but an inherent mischievousness. A #4 Cancer likes their protective shell, and many are happy working out of their home or car. A #12 Pisces likes to expand beyond their limitations and the place where they probably feel most comfortable is at the beach.

Beyond the dimensions, there is also the style of the places people prefer; colors, materials, traditional, contemporary or futuristic. Style is something that is shared by multiple Signs and described by what we call the four 'Elements'. In modern scientific terms, these are the four physical states of matter, which describe the transformation of nature.

A favorite example of the cycle of life that children learn quite early in school is the transformation of water. It is liquid in the ocean, that evaporates as a gas becoming clouds, falling to Earth as rain, hail or snow, becoming solid ice in the winter, then melting into streams, that reach rivers and return to the ocean to begin the cycle again.

There is a correlation between the Astrological Elements and states of matter. They are: Fire = Plasma, Earth = Solid, Air = Gaseous, Water = Liquid. The Element of a person's Sun reveals the preferred dimensions, while the Moon provides insights about their stylistic preferences.

If they have multiple Planets in an Element, that preference is enhanced. For example, a person with the Sun, Moon, Mercury and Venus in Aries, a Fire Sign, tends to want to live in a brightly lit Space.

Fortunately for them, there are two other Fire Signs, Leo and Sagittarius, who also like it on the bright side. So that Aries dominant person will find others who are comfortable sharing a Space with them.

The Wheel of the Signs with Their Elements

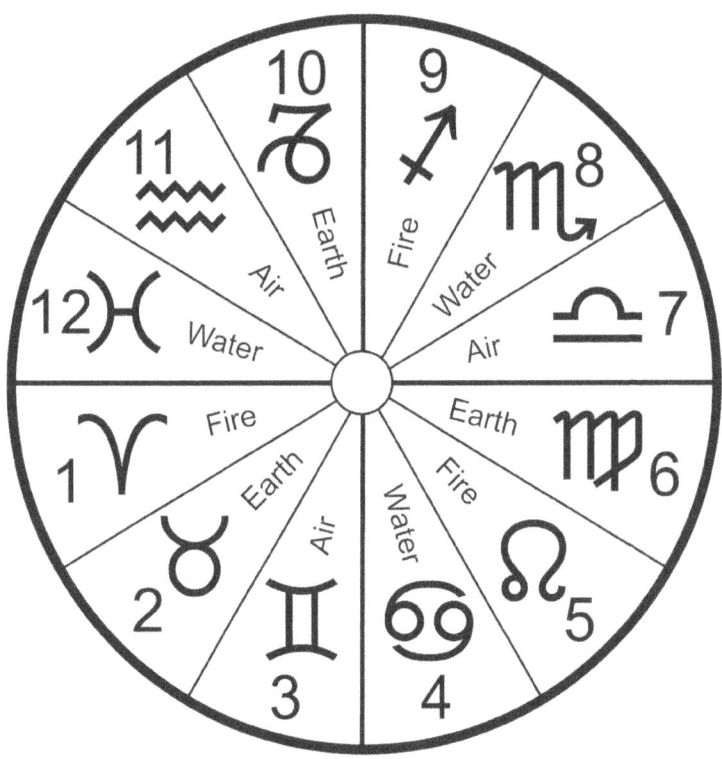

While having the Ascendant (Rising Sign) or the Moon in one of these Signs will filter a person's preferences, when it comes to size, the Sun Sign carries the biggest hammer. However, when it comes to what they expect in their professional workspace, the Signs of Jupiter and Saturn are strong indicators, because those Planets command the Space beyond the Earth's orbit.

Rather than pushing the influence of the Sun Sign aside, they fill in the other side of the picture of what people expect in their world. Sometimes, if the influence is at odds (opposed) to their personal program, it will show what that person will give up in their personal preferences to accommodate the needs of their work.

For example, a person with a Cancer Sun likes an intimate Space filled with comfortable objects, possessing emotional significance for them. But, if they have Saturn in the demanding, highly structured Sign of Capricorn they will push themselves outside of that comfort zone, into those high rises and office parks, because those surroundings equate to professional success for them. Because the work requires the denial of their comfort-loving self, they will make their home the epitome of the cozy little nest!

The Stylistic Preferences of the Elemental Triplicities

The Fire Signs: #1 Aries, #5 Leo and #9 Sagittarius. People with a Fire Sun position generally like larger Spaces than the Earth and Water Signs, but they not as expansive as the Air Signs. Fire likes to concentrate and then spread out in tendrils, so people with strong Fire in their Chart like their Spaces with a strong sense of purpose.

The Earth Signs: #2 Taurus, #6 Virgo and #10 Capricorn. They generally like larger Spaces than the Water Signs, but smaller Spaces than the Fire and Air Signs. They are inclined to surround themselves with natural materials, rather than high tech plastic and glass.

The Air Signs: #3 Gemini, #10 Libra and #11 Aquarius. These people require brighter Spaces than the other Signs, because they are very visual and social. They like to be aware of the spaces and the people around them.
Warning: There is an important factor to consider with the Air Signs. While they like lots of light and visual information in their living and working Spaces, they tend to be very light sensitive.

In a bedroom too much light, either electric, reflected or through a window can inhibit their ability to sleep well. This tends to be emphasized when a chart has multiple Planets in Air Signs.

♋   ♏   ♓

The Water Signs: #4 Cancer, #8 Scorpio and #12 Pisces. They generally like the smallest Spaces compared with the other Signs. Water is all about emotions so the way they feel about their surroundings matters a great deal. They like objects to which they have an emotional attachment, and when you see them get rid of something, realize there is probably a story, and maybe a tear connected to that.

The Twelve Signs and Their Spatial Preference

♈ ♂ #1 Aries the Ram is the Dynamic Sign of Mars and the original self-starters who tend to do best in the small Spaces. They like to personalize their domain and need a place to express their individuality, without much interference. That does not mean they can't share a Space. On the contrary, Fire Signs are social by nature. Strong willed Aries is happiest when they have someone to push against, especially when that person pushes back. Part of the secret here is that Aries has an almost psychic connection to their personal possessions and surroundings, a holdover from Pisces who precedes Aries in the circle of life. To be creative and happy they need to have their tools and touchstones handy.

So, while they like to share a Space, they need dominion over their personal tool chest. Being Mars ruled they tend to merge courage with a lack of experience, making them willing to venture into new Spaces, bringing their confidence with them. They will bring their environment with them through a favorite briefcase or bag, creating a very small halo of objects around themselves. You find strong Aries energy in many salespeople.

♉ ♀ #2 Taurus the Bull, as one of the Signs of Venus, is the most comfort inclined of the three Earth Signs, making them prefer intimate, personalized Spaces. Taurus is the Receptive Sign of Venus and it expresses the Venusian desire to feel safe and secure, maybe a little nested, and safely away from the traffic. Their work pace tends to be steady and consistent, so they like a Space where the colors are harmonious.

Understanding how clutter accumulates is very important for people with strong Taurus in their chart, because they like 'things'. They like to own objects, cars and property, because that makes them feel good, warm and content. Taurus the Bull tends to look down and that inclines a person to think about the past more than the future. With a Taurus Sun make sure that the scent of the place supports their personality.

♊ ☿ #3 Gemini the Twins likes their Spaces the smallest of the three Air Signs. Being the Dynamic Sign of mobile Mercury, they like to be close to doors and pathways. They do not like to be stuck in a corner away from everything that is happening. Of the three Air Signs, Gemini likes working closely with people and they are fine with sharing Spaces. Remember, they are the twins, who start their life sharing. They also like mirrors in their surroundings. It is not vanity, but visual playfulness that makes that de-Sign feature popular with the Twins. They like metal and glass, are very information dependent and require excellent light sources, otherwise they will complain.

Air and Water Signs are the two Most Extreme Elements When Comparing the Types and Sizes of the Spaces They Seek

♋ ☽ #4 Cancer the Crab, not surprisingly, likes smaller Spaces. Cancer is the Sign of the Moon, who affects the ocean's tides and women's cycles. That connection to the sea is epitomized by the Crab, who carries its personal shell around with them. Many Cancerians like to work out of their home or cars, which is a shell that moves around. They like comfort, which is more important to them than aesthetics. That doesn't mean they don't like beautiful things, but the emotional significance of an object is more important to them. They need the smell of the place to work for them, which is why they like their cars so much, it smells like their life, familiar.

People with multiple Planets in Cancer tend to accumulate things. There is something about the Cancer energy that encourages a poor posture, a natural tendency to curl up a little bit to protect their vulnerable belly. Designs that encourage a person to look down are the worst for promoting clutter, so choosing furnishings that encourage good posture is helpful in avoiding this pitfall.

♌ ☉ #5 Leo the Lion also likes to share a Space, if they like you, and is a bit more generous with sharing dominion than Aries. Leo is the Sign of the Sun, the center of attention, so Leo thrives on praise and the opportunity to be generous, which is why a small, isolated living or workspace starves their joy. While most people do better when they can command the Space (see the entrance from their 'throne'), and see what is going on around them, Leo equally needs to be seen. They like bright, colorful environments. They are naturally confident, so they have very little inclination towards accumulating clutter.

♍ ☿ #6 Virgo the Virgin, likes their Space a bit more roomy than the Bull but, more importantly they like close proximity with other people. This is the Receptive Sign of mobile Mercury, so they want to be closer to the pathways and need a bit of distraction and noise to keep them engaged. Being Mercury's Sign, they are information based, which makes them dependent on good light sources. On the flip side, it makes them sensitive to glare and noise. Like the

Dynamic Mercury Sign, Gemini, they like mirrors in their surroundings. People with strong Virgo in their charts must guard against taking organization into pathological territory. It comes out of their fear of being 'wrong'.

The Virgo time of year is the harvest, when a loss of valuable assets through lack of attention produces long-lasting repercussions, affecting the whole community. This anxious care of the details is why they call Virgos the perfectionists. Unlike Taurus, the Virgo energy tends to encourage good posture, so arranging the Space so their point of view promotes a 'heads up' attitude, will prevent any tendency to look down, which puts people into fear mode.

♎ ♀ #7 Libra the Scales prefers shared workspaces. They are the Dynamic Sign of Venus, so they tend to partner with others and rely upon that interaction to plot their path forward. Being higher in the sequence, they like a larger Space than Gemini, but they don't like a place that is too large, because it too easily becomes unbalanced, or out of scale with the furniture. Of the three Air Signs, Libra requires harmony the most.

Where Gemini is comfortable with activity and distraction, and Aquarius requires some chaos and alternative features to feel happy, Libra is very disrupted if the sounds, light sources and scents in their Space are discordant. While they are a responsive type of personality, due to their imperative to partner, they can be quite active and demanding when it comes to establishing harmony in their living and working Spaces.

♏ ♂ #8 Scorpio the Scorpion likes a more expansive Space than cozy Cancer. This is the Receptive Sign of Mars and Scorpions tend to impose strict boundaries, as they can be very territorial. For Scorpio, the question is about whether the Space is defensible. They do not like to spread out too much, because it means thinning out their defenses. Now and then Scorpio will be drawn to expansive Spaces with great views through extensive windows. That is the Eagle side coming out (Scorpio has four symbols, the scorpion, the snake, the eagle and the Phoenix). But when they move into the Space, they will find a well-insulated, protected, private nook to spend much of their time.

Watch out when you live with someone with strong Scorpio in their chart. In the depths of their souls they abhor clutter and when things get out of control, they are happy to redecorate with a gas can and a match. But, be hopeful, they can be persuaded to follow a gentler approach.

#9 Sagittarius the Centaur Archer. Of the three Fire Signs Sagittarius, the Centaur Archer, likes the largest, brightest Space, on par with the air Signs. It is the Dynamic Sign of Jupiter, the largest Planet, so like Aquarius, they like to have views of the world outside. Unlike Aquarius, they like to be closer to people and they are more willing to share Spaces. A unique feature of the Sagittarius personality is the desire for mobility.

They like lots of exits and opportunities to wander around beyond their normal environs. Sagittarius does not like to be contained and trying to put them in a small, constrained Space is a great way to find them perpetually absent. When someone bothers them, if they can't attack them, or charm them, then they put distance between them. You know something is really bothering a Sagittarius when you turn around and realize that they are suddenly gone!

#10 Capricorn the Sea Goat, unlike the other two Earth Signs, is a mythical creature. Capricorn is the Receptive Sign of Saturn with its many Moons and complex rings. That may be a hint about why Capricorn is drawn to extreme Spaces created by complex human cooperation. They seem drawn to the high rises and angular environments that Taurus abhors, and Virgo tolerates. The secret here is that Capricorn is ruled by Saturn which also rules Aquarius. This often creates unusual and modernistic tastes in living and working Spaces. Capricorn also likes the badges of power and prestige with a tendency to dark colors. If the Space is too comfortable and cozy, they may be concerned that they will be less productive.

#11 Aquarius, the Water Pourer needs the most amount of Space and the largest windows of the Air Signs. This is the Dynamic Sign of Saturn, so it is powerfully visual. The types and numbers of windows in a house that would prove problematic and distracting to most other Signs, works well for the Aquarians.

It is as if they were made to be outdoors in a vineyard, carrying their pitcher of water from stream to vines, scanning the rows, looking for plants in need of care. The Aquarian energy is seen as a guardian personality, so they tend to be broad viewers, who like the sense of living outside, so they are inclined to very modern, well-lit environments. Like Capricorn, they are drawn to large buildings. But they are very sensitive to electromagnetic fields, both natural and manufactured.

#12 Pisces the Fishes can be deceptive for a Water Sign. This is the Receptive Sign of grand Jupiter, and of the Water Signs they like the largest Spaces, like sea creatures. With Pisces, the boundaries between water and flesh often seem nebulous, making it hard to tell where their Space ends, and that of others begins. Being a mutable Sign, they are the most social of the Water Signs and they seem to be natural over lappers.

They easily move into another person's Space, like a big house cat, fitting into the unused nook. Even when they occupy a large Space, they will often create a small haven for their personal dreaming. People with strong Pisces in their charts are not very attached to 'things'. Because of that they can accumulate 'stuff' because they forget that it is theirs.

As you consider how to make your surroundings more effective, do not let your Sun Sign, or those of people who share the Space, stop you from using solid design principles. A great deal of what makes a Space work are ergonomics, light sources and practicalities. But knowing the size and style of the domain that your Sun Sign is happiest with, is a wonderful way to use extra insights to personalize your perfect Space.

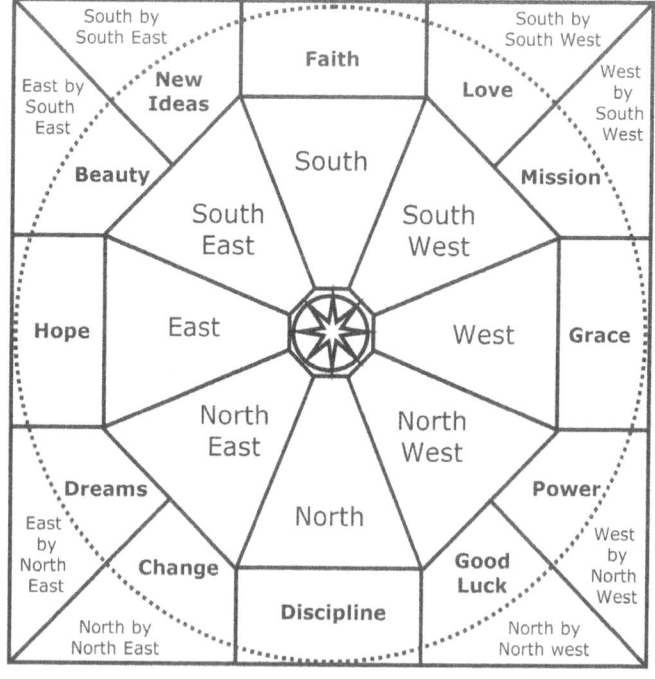

The Meaning of the Compass Directions

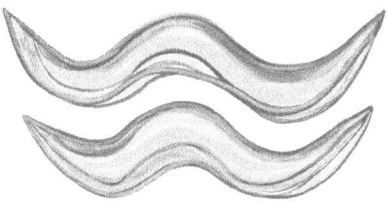

Chapter Eleven: The Secret Power in Local Space Charts

The Horizon Chart or Local Space Chart (LSC) is different from what most people are familiar with. The classic Astrology Chart is a map of where the Planets are located in the sky, at a particular moment, as they travel along the Ecliptic. It includes references to where the Ecliptic crosses the Eastern (Ascendant) and Western (Descendant) Horizons, and where it crosses the highest (MC) and lowest (IC) points in that celestial circle. *See the meaning of the compass directions opposite.*

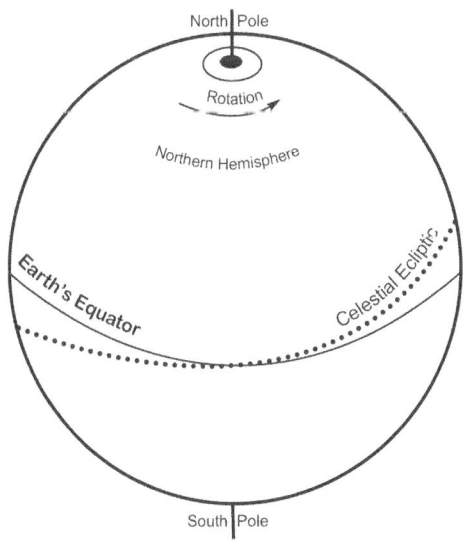

The Horizon Chart, which is equally ancient, marks the line of sight directions to the Planets from where the Chart is centered. It is used almost exclusively for birth Charts.

Essentially it tells us how a person has been programmed to prefer certain directions by those grand electromagnetic transmitters we call the Planets. For a quick example, if we know that Jupiter was rising in the Southeast when a person was born, we expect them to encounter Jovian experiences in that direction. They'll be drawn to a college in that direction.

The Personal Horizon or Local Space Chart

America USA
Natal Chart
Jul 4 1776
5:10 PM LMT +5:00:39
Philadelphia
39N57 08 075W09 51

The Horizon Chart can be calculated by many of the prevalent Astrological programs, so it has become a common, although underused tool in three-dimensional Astrology. The problem is that most Astrologers don't know what to do with these Charts.

The modern Local Space Chart software road into town on the popular coattails of **AstroCartography**, a system which produces an easy to understand world map showing where the Planets were overhead at the time of the Chart. It offers personal insights about which states, and countries would offer the best, or worst experiences for the Native.

The AstroCartography Chart

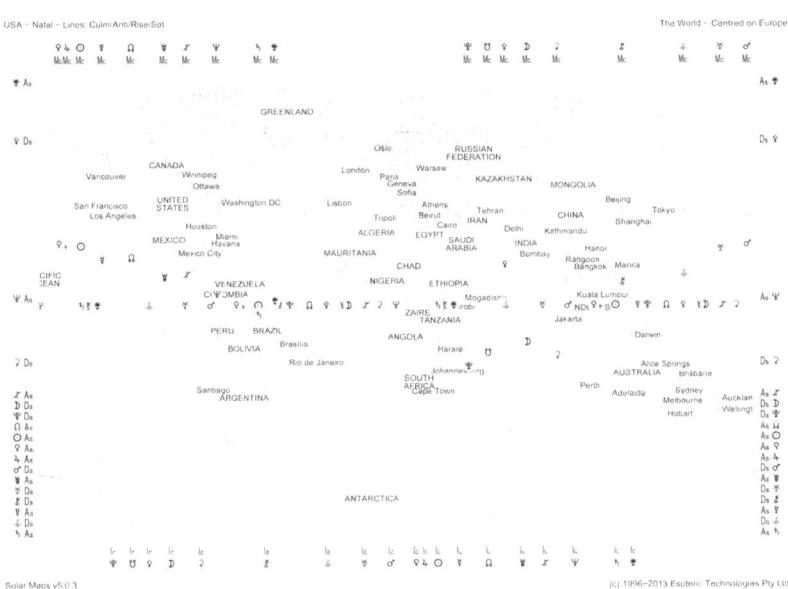

In comparison Horizon Charts are up close and personal and typically people place a transparency of the Horizon Chart on a map, with your home at the center. Then you look for places along their lines related to each Planet's energy. When we first learned about Horizon Charts the speaker mentioned that when they traveled to work, coincidentally along their Neptune line, they had a hard time staying awake at the wheel. One of their most memorable suggestions was that you could always find a good hair salon along your Venus line. Cool! But the reality is that these days you'll find a hairdresser by asking your girlfriend and then use online reviews for everything else.

So, rather than being a helpful tool, the LSC is treated mostly as a 'fun to play with' astrological oddity. Admittedly, it works, which demonstrates that Astrology is valid, but we already know that! Considering the ancient and revered history of Horizon Charts, being used for aligning important buildings and Sacred Sites, it is ridiculous that it has such limited utility today.

That happened because the Astrologer mathematicians who revived the system were not Geomancers, so they were not fluent in the language of environmental 'magic', physics, or Feng Shui. There is a better and more personally powerful way to use Horizon Charts, in homes and workplaces, to improve your daily life, that we've used in our environmental Astrology practice for the last couple of decades.

Instead of putting the map on the house or office, put it on you! Treat your body like what it is, a radio receiver for numerous frequencies, including many beyond your conscious awareness. Your main antennae are the Chakras on the front of your body, running from the base of your torso to your hairline. When your turn yourself to face a transmitting Planet, you are tuning into its unique message.

We theorize that your aura is programmed at birth by the unique electromagnetic power of the Planets arrayed in the sky around you. Imagine your aura as a balloon, at birth the messages coming from the Planets sprayed brightly colored stripes of energy on the surface. Even when your aura expands, that pattern remains for the rest of your life, filtering your perception of those compass directions. So yes, when you look in the direction where Venus was at your birth, you are seeing the world through rose colored glasses.

The best place to start doing this is at your desk, because when you tune into the correct station for your desired purpose, the results are quickly forthcoming. The key is selecting a suitable broadcast station for the activity. When you tune into Mars for your sales calls, you're putting some extra spark in your belly.

If you face Jupiter when you make your travel plans you open your mind to far off places and choose optimism over anxiety. When you face Pluto or Neptune during meditation or yoga beware, because that can produce trans-dimensional experiences, obsessive in the former and boundless in the later.

We've noticed that successful people instinctively arrange their workspaces to face their most productive Planets. A client who ran her own marketing company set up her desk to face her Jupiter, a good choice for an enterprise all about expanding the client's sales. But, when her children called, she pivoted her chair to face her Moon, the Planet of nurturing and food. When her girlfriends called, she turned towards her Venus line, the Planet of sharing, pleasures and cooperation.

If you are like many of our clients, your 'comfy chair' faces either your Moon or Venus, the comfort Planets. Your most productive reading and writing chair probably faces your Mercury, although if you lean towards philosophical topics, you probably prefer Jupiter. Craft people's work tables often face Mercury, hairdresser's favorite station often has them facing Venus, and computer game designers like to face Uranus.

Transferred executives who feel like they've lost their mojo, have gotten stuck at a new desk facing an ineffective Planetary direction. The human body makes a wonderful dowsing rod. That's why successful people trust their feelings. So, if you change workplaces and your previous level of success is eluding you, turn your desk around until it feels like you're facing your 'Lucky Stars' again.

Bosses and business owners prefer to face their Sun, Jupiter or Mars. Accountants seek out Saturn or Mercury, depending on whether they are conservative or innovative in their style. If one of those Planets is in Libra, the Scales, that may take priority. When people feel unplugged, they are often facing an empty zone. If they feel confused or overwhelmed, they may be facing their Uranus, Neptune or Pluto because those messages are hard to turn towards practical applications.

When you face salespeople towards their Mercury or Mars, they are more effective, although those selling beauty and skin related products do well facing their Venus. Going from desk to desk to improve the performance of a team facing challenges, being cognizant of how they are seeing each other, is a great way helping them get back on track, or more accurately, get better aligned.

Remember that your Smart phone has a compass app, so arrive early to business meetings to select the seat that works best for you and the task. For first time sales, facing your bold Mars is great, but if patient negotiation and cooperation is the goal, then face your Venus or Saturn. Lecture facing Mercury or Jupiter. At the casinos, face Mercury, Jupiter or a dash of Uranus depending on how wild an experience you want.

When you go house hunting, if you are facing your Moon when you walk in the front door, you will probably buy the place because it will feel like home. Performers love stages where they face their Sun, Moon or Jupiter, and dislike those that face Saturn or Uranus, although the latter can be exciting, if unpredictable.

The key with Horizon Charts and Astro*Carto*Graphy is to integrate your insights from the Natal Chart, because an Extrovert of Introvert Planet, according to the Table of Rulerships* (see figure), acts that way in a Location Chart. For greater success in the outside world, a person will do better facing their aggressive Natal Mars in Rulership (Aries or Scorpio), instead of their internally focused Jupiter in Detriment (Gemini or Virgo), which could instead promote their inner development. With Astro*Carto*Graphy people make this mistake, moving to their Venus Line, expecting all wine and roses, but forgetting that their Detriment Venus in Scorpio is more inclined to obsession than commitment. Moving to their Ruling Mars in Scorpio line instead would help them find love on their own terms.

Notes for the Advanced Astrologer

The Natal compass directions rule; True North works better than magnetic, because the body knows where the Ecliptic is, since it is the direction of the light and warmth. When you move to a different city you don't relocate the Local Space Chart.

Curiously people often improve their material success by facing their Part of Fortune, which implies that the Parts are directional rather than psychological. Chinese Astrology has a similar time-honored technique, for calculating your lucky direction. You start with the angular clockwise distance from the Sun to Jupiter, then apply that angle clockwise from the Imum Coeli.

The technique shows the Asian preference for an Earth based system, using the IC, or ground beneath your feet as the important reference. Modern Western Astrology tends to be sky centered! Clearly there are many ways to use Horizon Charts, and we hope you find this technique helpful. Remember, by facing the correct direction, you are choosing the Planet that will be your champion!

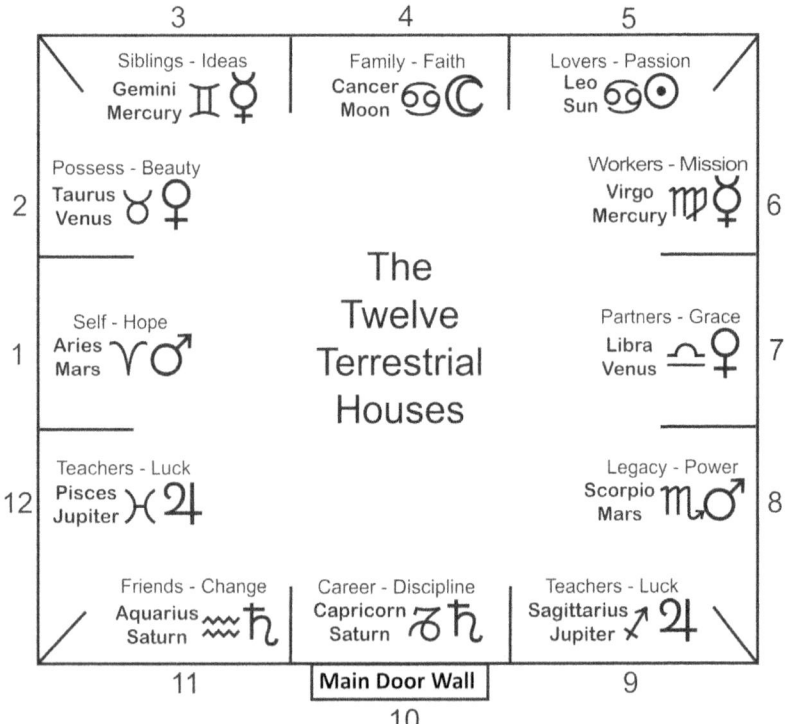

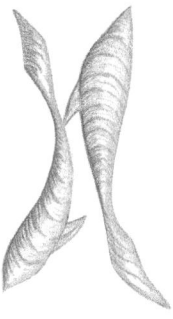

Chapter Twelve: Calendrical Healing

This is the first part of a three-chapter segment that explores Astrological Healing. This first chapter explains the Environmental Healing System (EHS) built into the Planetary Calendar. The next chapter is a deeper look at the Essential Oils that are used in the system. The third chapter explains the 'Terrestrial Houses' that determine where the Meditation and Essential Oils are used.

The EHS was created to work with the Planetary Calendar because the recommended actions are timed to the Lunations. With each New and Full Moon, the Calendar provides a suggested meditation and an Essential Oil recommendation that was created based on the theme in that Lunation's unique Chart.

Note: While the calendar's meditations are carefully crafted based on the entire Chart, creating one for any Lunation is simple; consider the primary actions of the Signs involved and express how that acts in your life most effectively.

In Astrology, location matters, so the Meditations and the Essential Oils are used in specific spots in the home. That location is determined by where the Signs of the Lunation fall in the Twelve Terrestrial Houses (TTH). The TTH is an environmental map that we've used for many years, based on the Western Astrological Houses and the Asian Feng Shui Bagua, with some insightful innovations from modern Kinesiology. The calendar and day planner contain basic instructions for using the EHS for clearing energetic debris, but we are exploring it here so you can apply it more creatively towards your personal goals. Nothing supercharges spiritual connections like creativity, except maybe love.

Healing Environmental Scars

Transits can adversely affect the physical and energetic condition of both the person's aura and their living spaces. In response, people may restrict their movements, physical and emotional, to stay in a 'pain free zone'.

This healing technique works by engaging the person mentally through the Meditation, emotionally through the Essential Oils and physically through activating sections of their surroundings. When challenging Transits, big and small, bulldoze their way through a person's Chart, those scars are stored in the aura and the personal Twelve Terrestrial Houses.

The TTH is where the Astrological Houses come down to Earth from the heavens and land in your home. This is an Earth-based perspective, looking down on our living spaces, rather than gazing up at the Stars. The EHS systematically clears those zones in both the person's aura and their Terrestrial Houses, hopefully restoring more flexibility to life.

While sweeping a space with sage smoke clears the recent life static in a current or new home, it doesn't dislodge those deeper scars that connect you to your surroundings. The EHS does that deeper cleaning by using the tidal force of the Lunations, brought into focus with the Meditations and supercharged with an energetic boost from the Essential Oils, precisely placed in the Terrestrial Houses related to that Sun/Moon pair.

We've had clients whose lives were so hemmed in by thorns left by past Transits, that they traveled through life as if they were on train tracks, stuck on a set path without options. That is why moving to a new home can be a liberating experience, a person can discard the furniture and objects tied to a painful past.

The aura is like a computer hard drive and the Terrestrial Houses are like an attached backup drive. Even when you do the personal work to clear the aura, the memory of what you've cleared is still stored in your couch, your desk, or that dark, domineering armoire that towers over the bed.

The advantage of using the EHS is that it reformats both memories, ensuring that you won't imprint the newly cleared space with those old files. This is helpful in both your current home and when you move to a new home.

The method is simple. During the New or Full Moon, with a pen, write down the meditation from the calendar, adding your personal intentions. Get a small bowl of water and add a total of twenty to thirty drops of the suggested Essential Oils. As an alternative you can use a diffuser instead.

Ideally, place the Meditation and the Essential oils in the area of the recommended Terrestrial House, where you will see and smell them, while saying the Meditation out loud. Then meditate on that subject for a short time to put you in tune with the message of that Lunation, adding your own intentions.

If the life issues related to that Terrestrial House are very important to you, between then and the next Lunation, periodically go to the spot and refresh the Oils, repeating the Mediation.

Generally, we suggest a single Essential Oil for the New Moon and a blend of two or three for the Full Moon. The choice of the Terrestrial House highlighted is based on the position of the Sun, but for the Full Moon you can add the opposite House for the position of Luna.

It is helpful to make a copy of the meditation and put some drops of the Essential Oils on the corner of the paper. Tape it to the mirror where you get dressed and read it first thing in the morning. Place it so it is between the height of your heart and the height of your eyes. Gradually, the scent will fade, as will your tendency to repeat the Meditation, along with the residual negativity in that area of your life.

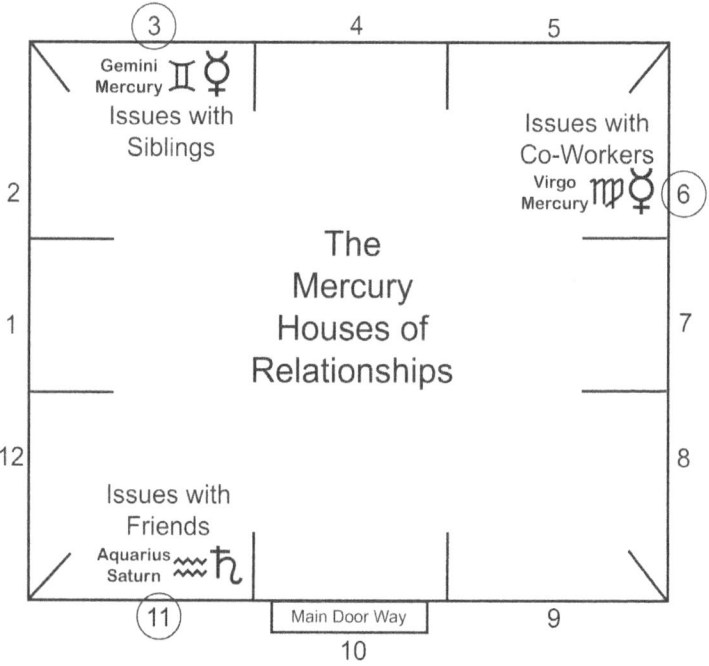

For example, if you had difficult issues with siblings, that is a Third House, Gemini affair. During the New and Full Moon, when the Sun is in Gemini, the third Terrestrial House in your home is highly active, it is also where your aura stores those memories.

If you feel like you're not getting enough love in your life, there are several lunations whose tidal currents you can ride. If it's the sensual pleasures of love, then the Second House and the Taurus Lunations work best. For heart-warming romance, the

Fifth House and the Leo Lunations are where and when to focus on that. If it's commitment and a soul merging relationship that you're interested in, then the Seventh House and the Libra Lunations are the key.

By infusing the power of that Lunar tide with your Intentional Mediations, and boosting them with the Essential Oils, you can wash away those scars at a deep level. Do the steps at least three times near the Lunation and if you wish, you can repeat the steps every day, stopping two days before the next Lunation, because the next tidal message will be on its way.

Next we will explore how Astrology and Herbs work together, especially Essential Oils, abbreviated E.O., because that's the energetic tool we use in the Calendar's system.

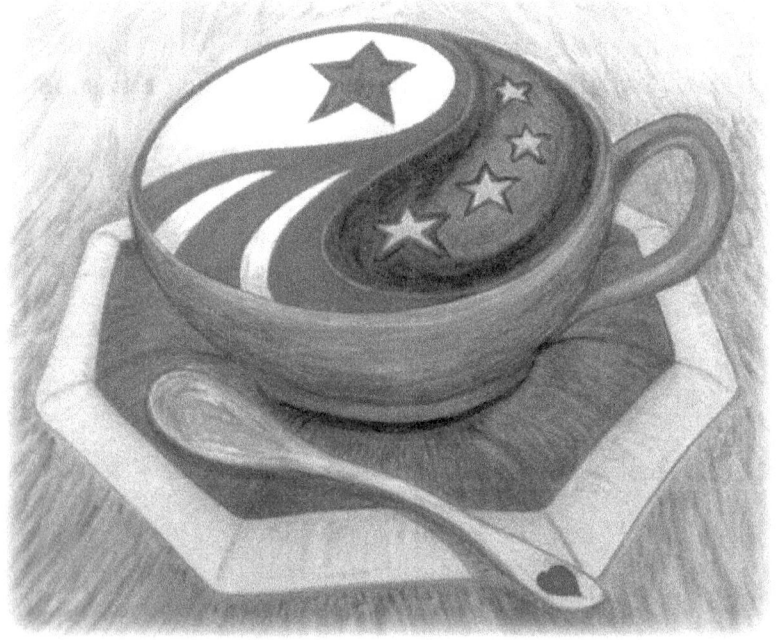

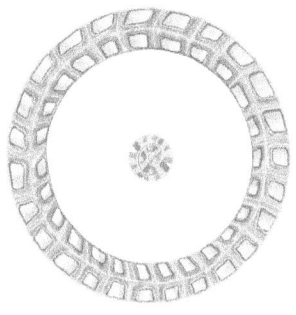

Chapter Thirteen: Essential Oils as Astrological Tools

The Essential Oils extracted from plants are wonderful healing tools because they are familiar, delightful and humans have no barriers against the power of scent. Exploring them in relation to Astrology is also a wonderful way to connect sensually with the themes of the Planets and Signs.

Astrology and herbs have been linked since ancient times, with some of the greatest reference books about assignments being those connecting medicinal plants to the Planets. As you delve into this system, called the Planetary Signatures, the similarities are pretty obvious; red hot peppers connected to the red Planet Mars, lavender flowers, whose name's means 'to clean', linked with Mercury, seductive Jasmine aligned with Venus, the heart-warming rose being dear to the Sun and belly warming garlic reflecting the Moon.

Just one example of the scientific confirmation for this is the established fact that rose oil vibrates at the same frequency as the human heart. We also see the symbolic relationship that exists between the Sun and Moon among plants; Solar Cacao, the source of heart-warming chocolate, lives symbiotically with "La Madre de Cacao". That Lunar plant provides protective shade and its falling, chemical-rich leaves protect the cacao from invasive insects.

> Indian Astrologers call Sol and Luna
> "the two eyes of the Universe" and their
> separation is what gives us perspective.

While spicy ginger would seem related to Mars, because its warmth is healing, its applications flexible, its nature exotic and it travels well, it's in the domain of Jupiter. Sandalwood is a woody resin that protects the tree from insects by filling bore holes. The scent of Sandalwood enhances meditation and it's used in the grand stone churches where people seek protection, which exemplifies serious, solemn Saturn. Long before our current system of taxonomy, Astrologer Herbalists classified plants with the Planetary Signatures, because they describe the plant's healing action.

Here is a quick look. Sun herbs benefit the heart. Moon herbs help the tummy. Mercury herbs calm the nervous system. Venus herbs balance the hormones and minerals. Mars herbs heat the blood and hormones. Jupiter herbs strengthen the muscles. Saturn herbs fortify the bones.

Essential Oils

What are Essential Oils? They are volatile compounds from the plant's defensive and hormonal systems, that are extracted by either cold pressing, steam distillation or chemical solvents. The Essential Oils we use for environmental healing come from plants. Many destroy harmful pathogens like bacteria, viruses and fungi when added to cleaning water or through diffusion in the air and those invaders never develop of resistance to Essential Oils. Some promote good feelings, social harmony and of course romance, which explains the massive size of the perfume industry. Unfortunately, many commercial scents depend on synthetic ingredients to give them staying power.

The power of the Essential Oils comes from the areas they affect. The senses of smell and taste are different from the so called 'higher' senses of sight and hearing, which are located close to the frontal brain. In the frontal cortex the signals from your eyes and ears are interpreted. What they receive is very different from what is projected on the screen of your consciousness.

In comparison, the senses of smell and taste ascend through the parts of the brain related to emotions and spatial memory. These two senses are inextricably linked. Eventually they pass through the conscious mind, ending up in the non-verbal, right brain where creativity and intuition live.

That is why a scent stimulates an emotion and may remind you of a place. Because it goes through the speech centers, it can rob you of the ability to formulate words, leaving you literally speechless, left with only visual thinking. That's why it so hard to verbally describe a taste. The current idea that there are only five flavors may come from the difficulty people have finding words to describe what their palates are experiencing.

Because that primary area where scent and taste travel are in the ancient parts of the brain, you never forget a scent and it is always tied to an emotion. This is important in healing because to make a profound change in a person's attitude, it's not enough to convince the conscious brain, or even the higher consciousness. You also need to reach deep into the emotions. But, the Essential Oils reach beyond the emotional body.

That's because Essential Oils carry a beneficial electrical charge, which raises the frequency wherever they are used. They are especially helpful in Calendrical Healing because they dissipate with time, allowing the focus to easily shift to the adjoining Terrestrial House at the next Lunation. When a person keeps focusing on the same issue again and again and again, that's obsession. They are not letting life flow. Read the Chapter about the Chinese Elements to understand the importance of movement in healing.

Besides being placed in a bowl of water, Essential Oils mixed with water can also be diffused or sprayed. You can scent a sachet or add it to your washing water. If you incorporate that same Essential Oil into a perfume, bath oil or spray for your sheets or furniture, you can massively magnify the beneficial effect every time you experience them.

Your choice of Essential Oils can also augment your personal qualities. For example: A person born with the Sun in Leo who feels that they need to strengthen their sense of love, could diffuse the oil Rose Bulgaria in their bedroom.

People who feel they need greater mental clarity often use Lavender, a Mercury herb, however, its side effect is that it promotes chastity, something it shares with the crystal Amethyst. If no EO on your Sign list appeals to you, look at your Moon or Ascendant Sign. Alternately, consider those connected to the Sign that shares the same Planet Ruler. For example: A person born with the Sun in Libra, Capricorn Rising and the Moon in Scorpio, who doesn't like the scent of the very Venusian Ylang Ylang, might do better with the Taurus oils of Jasmine or Bergamot, which also connect to Capricorn and Scorpio. Sometimes you just need to stick your nose into the blend and see how it makes you feel!

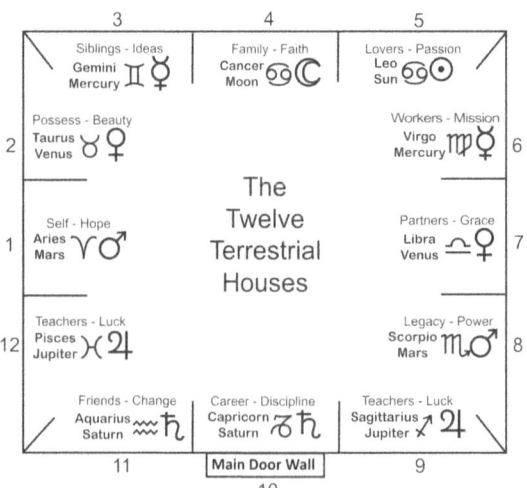

The Essential Oils in the Terrestrial Houses

Because we are using these Essential Oils for the Environmental Healing Technique, we are categorizing them by the Twelve Terrestrial Houses. Each House relates to a Sign and the Planet that is its Extrovert Expression, or in 'traditional speak', the Ruler.

The First House, Aries, Mars: Use oils that promote courage, reduce anxiety and enforce effective boundaries. Mars oils heat and activate. The mints arouse the senses, stimulate circulation and soothe digestion. The most potent and popular is Peppermint, but don't forget gentler spearmint, which can also be used as a Mercury scent. Red Mandarin Orange and Bergamot, both citrus oils, work well here and in the Martial Eighth House.

Second House, Taurus, Venus: Because this area relates so strongly to the senses of smell and taste, the oils used here have a great deal of influence. Jasmine is a very seductive scent that empowers your feminine side and promotes the appreciation of beauty. Ylang Ylang is an aphrodisiac flower with a high romantic energy. Vanilla is the quintessential Taurus herb because it is appealing in so many applications.

The Third House, Gemini, Mercury: Lemon, Lime and Neroli are all good for the nervous system and work well here. Thyme lifts the spirits, balances the nervous system and brings a lightness and mental brightness to your life. Lavender, which is more at home in the 6th House also works here, but not if you are encouraging flirting, which is a third House thing.

The Fourth House, Cancer, Moon: Roman Chamomile works in both the 4th and 5th Houses. Geranium is very nurturing. Rose Geranium brings that to another 'love level'. Marjoram promotes strong, stable femininity. Neroli, which is a Mercury oil, also works well here by dissolving grief and worry. Vanilla, which is a Venus oil can also be used here effectively, blended with a touch of Lemon or Orange. Many of these oils are also balancers of hormones so they are especially effective in the feminine house of the Moon.

The Fifth House, Leo, Sun: Rose is an aphrodisiac that promotes love, joy and passion in your life. It smells very different in the bottle from you might expect, so start of slowly with small amounts and then adjust. Pink Grapefruit is the most Solar of the citrus oils. It lifts the spirits and brings a sweet lightness to your outlook. Helichrysum is fortifying to the heart, it brings enthusiasm and joy to your day. Orange and Lemon also work well in this House, to lift the mood and clear the mind.

The Sixth House, Virgo, Mercury: Lavender (especially Lavandula Agustifolia) is very soothing and promotes gentle social interactions. It encourages mental clarity and attention to detail and duty. Rosemary strengthens your intuitive self and improves your mental awareness of those messages. The milder members of the mint family; Spearmint and Catnip would also serve concerns of this House well.

Seventh House, Libra, Venus: Sage and Cedar both suit this House well. As does the Jasmine, Ylang Ylang and Vanilla that are so comfortable in the Second House. That is because this is an area that does well with blends, so Bergamot, which is used in the Mars Houses, also blends wonderfully here, in small amounts. Even woody oils like Pine or Eucalyptus would fit in a seventh House blend, if you especially intended to formalize or stabilize a relationship.

The Eighth House, Scorpio, Mars: Cinnamon has the red color expected in a Mars oil, with the potent seductiveness that appeals to Scorpio. It lifts the spirits, warms the body, boosts the energy and relieves fatigue, improves your sense of well-being, emotional accessibility and confidence. Red Mandarin Orange and Bergamot, both citrus oils, also work well here. Clove Bud boosts the energy from the root chakra up, helping you tap into your primal power.

The Ninth House, Sagittarius, Jupiter: Ginger and most of the citrus oils, especially Orange and Bergamot work well here. Oregano extends your horizons and maximizes your sense of optimism. Two twelfth House oils that also work well are Frankincense and Patchouli. The first helps in mediation while the second is an exotic, magical aphrodisiac that promotes male potency. The secret with Patchouli is to blend it in small amounts with either Bergamot or Frankincense.

The Tenth House, Capricorn, Saturn: This is a highly structured House, so the wood oils work best, such as Pine Needle, Sandalwood, Cedar with Vanilla. Because these resins are heavy scents you can blend them, preferably with a citrus which will help balance and effectively volatize them.

The Eleventh House, Aquarius, Saturn: This area does well with strong and sometimes unusual scents. Clary Sage is a gentle euphoric that balances the aura and clears confusion. Eucalyptus gets the winds of change flowing through your mind and your destiny. Tea Tree stimulates positive, serious change.

The Twelfth House, Pisces, Jupiter: Frankincense aids in meditation and brings a greater sense of spiritual connection. Myrrh has a sensual sweetness with a spiritual sensitivity. Sandalwood works well here and in the Tenth House. Patchouli is another Jupiter floral that works well here in small amounts.

Some Tips for Using Essential Oils

Warning: Keep the oils away from the eyes, nose and skin. If you do get oils someplace you shouldn't, flush the area with milk (dairy or nut) or oil, NOT WATER, which will potentiate it! Anything fatty will neutralize it.

Don't hold the bottle to your nose because eventually you will get it on your skin. Besides that not being a good idea, the residual scent will interfere with your ability to smell any other scents.

Instead, put a drop or two on a scent stick, wave it around a little bit to allow it to volatize and then smell it. When we blend, we wear disposable latex gloves. They protect the skin and they will not absorb the scent as your bare fingers would.

If we were making a three-oil blend, working with five or six possible Essential Oils, we would lay out a line of scent sticks, writing the name of one oil at the end of each stick and then putting a drop of that oil on the other end. Now can we hold the potential EO sticks side by side and smell them together, being careful to not cross contaminate them. This gives us a sense of what they will smell like when blended.

We may prefer more of one oil than another in a blend, and we can simulate that by how far away we hold a stick from the nose. This doesn't give you the complete story, because when the chemicals interact the overall scent changes. Once we have our potential blend, we'll put a single drop of each into a small bottle, or preferably a washable glass dish and give them time to get to know each other. Then we'll see how the scent changes. Now we can adjust the proportion of the ingredients by adding drops, until we have a formula we like.

Two Helpful Tips: First, keep good notes, so if the blend turns out great you can reproduce the formula.

Second, sometimes a blend doesn't work out, that's okay! But, that why washable glass bowls are a good idea; it's hard and sometimes close to impossible to get the scent out of those little bottles. It's better to use them once the formula is set. The one-ounce size is best; add ten to twenty drops of the blended oils and fill it up with water.

For a perfume we use alcohol. For a massage oil mix it in a wide mouth jar and use very small amounts of EO; the scent should be evident, but not even close to overwhelming, because too much can irritate the skin, so err on the side of caution.

A well-balanced EO blend has three notes. A base note from a resin or wood. A middle note from an herbal or floral. A top note made from a lighter floral or citrus. This aligns with the trilogy of the physical, emotional and mental/spiritual. It also aligns with the Ascendant, the Moon and Mercury/Sun. Here are some examples of blends. 1) Sandalwood, Ylang Ylang, Pink Grapefruit 2) Pine, Spearmint, Lemon 3) Frankincense, Rose, Lavender 4) Cedar, Jasmine, Orange. 5) Vanilla, Neroli, Lemon.

When energetically charging a Terrestrial House use either a bowl of water or a diffuser. Store the Essential Oils away from direct sunlight and extreme temperature. Citrus oils last one to two years, florals about five and resins up to ten. Their longevity varies depending on quality. Of course, they don't last that long if you use enough of them to make a difference!

Make sure they are natural oils and not synthetics, such as candle oils and commercial air sprays. With some of the expensive oils like Rose, Ylang Ylang and Jasmine, it is common for companies to mix them with a neutral base oil. This has the advantage of packaging them in a larger, easier to handle bottle, that is also more reasonably priced. The scent matters, but so does the frequency, so buy good oils to get better results. Now let's look at where to put those Essential Oils!

The 12 Terrestrial Houses

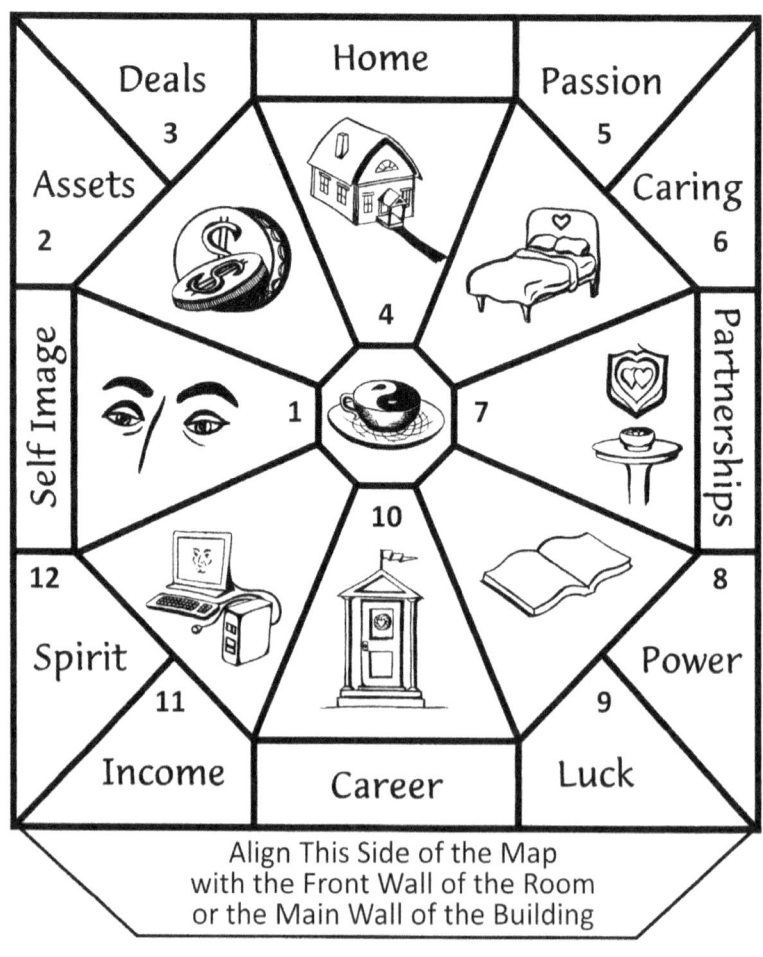

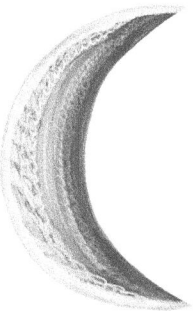

Chapter Fourteen: The Twelve Terrestrial Houses

This chapter explains how to apply the twelve Astrological Houses to your home and workplace, in a form we call the Terrestrial Houses. This principle was adapted from modern versions of Feng Shui, where the pattern of the cosmos is brought down to Earth and into your home. We will explain how, by changing what you have in your Terrestrial Houses, you plot a different path on the map of your life.

We also introduce a three-part healing system that we built into the Planetary Calendar for sequentially clearing energetic debris from your life. In our many years of writing and teaching we have found this subject the hardest to communicate, because understanding how our surroundings function is an experiential knowledge that people react to automatically from the unconscious parts of the brain. Rather than belaboring you with the philosophy, we are going to jump pretty quickly to the action steps, because that is where this will make sense.

Numerous cultures have energetic maps to be used on the Earth. In Feng Shui it's called the Bagua, which has eight parts. We call our map the Twelve Terrestrial houses. All these were initially aligned with the compass directions, but Asia Astrologers recognized that they could be applied inside rooms and houses irrespective of the magnetic directions. That's because, due to the design of the body, people have clearly defined kinesiological responses to building interiors, which in their raw form can be seen in the fight or flight reactions.

The Asian Bagua

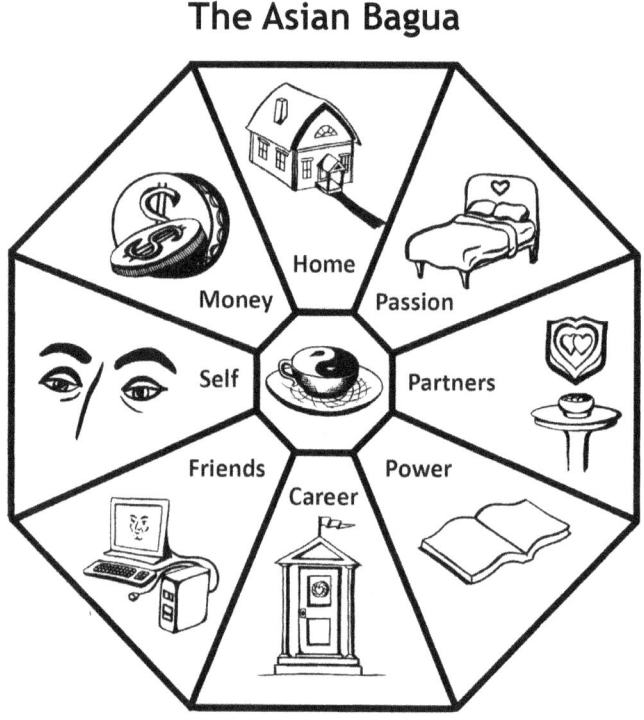

We react to our surroundings based on how and where we feel vulnerable and how we plan to keep ourselves safe. When we feel the need for salvation we look up. Why? Because climbing a tree or getting to high ground is wired into our anatomy as a safety strategy!

The twelve energy fields that we call the Signs, are part of the electrical and physical body's design. To understand the world the body interactively projects this pattern onto the surroundings in twelve clearly defined regions. Because it is an interactive relationship, a person's life can be read from their space and conversely, changes in those surroundings stimulate transformations in the person's life.

The Nature of Yin and Yang in the Bagua

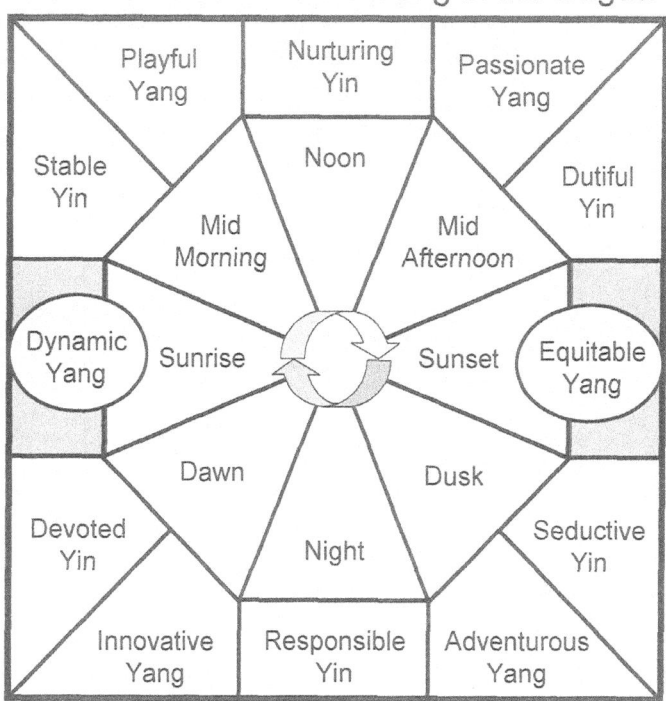

In a celestial Chart, when a Planet is in a Sign, and in a House, it is Actor with a Role who makes things happen in a Place. If the pattern we project around us is composed of the twelve Terrestrial Houses, it only takes a small imaginative stretch to think of your favorite chair, or a piece of art, or a pretty crystal as a Planet and by moving objects you are re-arranging your Terrestrial Houses. Why not? You an expression of the universe!

When you look around you how people live synergistically with their surroundings; stressful events manifest as clutter, while falling in love turns into homes filling up with flowers. Because it is interactive, you can let the magic happen by making actual, or even symbolic changes, that will stimulate changes in your life.

Let's say you have a tall, imposing piece of wooden furniture sitting in the Number Five romance section. That big piece of lumber sounds a lot like Saturn, and if your love life and sense of joy has been restricted and crunched by authority issues, maybe you're ready for a transit. Let's move that Saturn out of your love life and into the Number Ten Career Section, where she belongs. You'll get a bit more sparkle in your eyes and others will take you more seriously at work too.

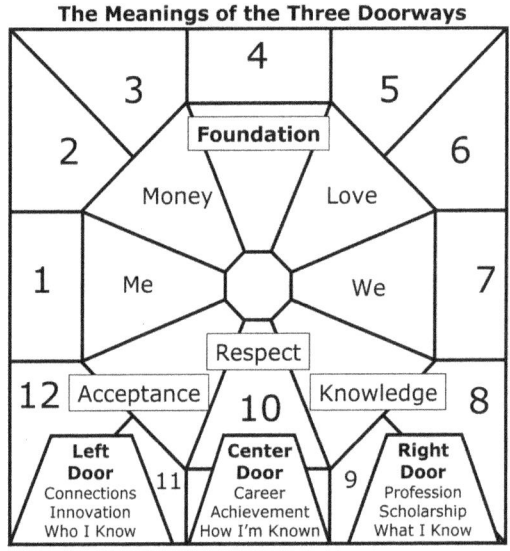

Accepting dominion over your space and recognizing that the imbalances there are not part of your authentic self, is the first step making the debris dissolve and the and joy bloom.

The Calendrical Healing system

Here is the Planetary Calendar system for systematically clearing the twelve Terrestrial Houses of obstructive, energetic debris. The steps are performed on the New and Full Moons. Each Lunation has a unique meditation, and an Essential Oils suggestion that is placed in a specific Terrestrial House. The steps can be done anytime during the two and a half days when the Lunation is active. If an area of your life needs more attention, make sustaining improvements there; a lamp, a piece of symbolic artwork or an energized crystal chosen for the Planet you want to see Transiting that House.

People often have a hard time aligning the map. The key question is this; what part of your body is closest to the parts of the room? Learn by doing! Pick a rectangular room with one door. Walk in and stop inside the doorway. Know this, your left side is vulnerable, while the right side is your strength. Point at the far left-hand corner with your left hand. That is the area of talents and money, that which you want to protect. Point at the far-right corner with your right-hand. That is the area of passion and love which you want to share.

The near half of the room relates to Houses Eight through Twelve, for the social life. The far half of the room relates to Houses two through six, which is the personal life. In the middle of the left wall is the Ascendant, the First House and the sense of self. Opposite that on the right wall is the Seventh House of marriage. Just remember, what matters is how the space relates to your body.

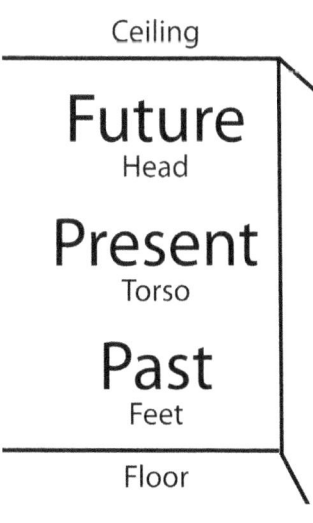

The map is not only horizontal, but also vertical. The lower third (legs) represents your past, the middle third (torso) is your present and the upper third (shoulders and head) is your future. Address current issues at the same height as your belly and upper chest. Changes that are too high place your good in the future. Normally trying to change the past is an iffy pursuit, but rearranging the lower sections of the room can help you change your attitude about those experiences.

More Hints on Seasonal Oil Placements

Consistently placing the Oils at the Lunations is appropriate for public spaces, especially meditation or yoga centers, because the rush of people disrupt their balance. Guard against saturating the air of your personal surroundings with Essential Oils, because they will overwrite the natural living scents that your body depends on for a sense of home. Use the Oils in small amounts, so they stay localized in the chosen section and infuse them with intention. Essential Oils can be toxic and irritating so treat them carefully, keeping them away from the eyes, nose and mouth.

For the Full Moon use at least two Oils in a blend, because they balance the opposing Sun and Moon positions. The New Moon can use one. The placement is based on the Sun, although at the Full Moon an option would be to use the two polarities.

For example, when the Sun is in Leo and the Moon is Full in Aquarius, we would place the blend in House Number Five for Leo the heart. A good choice for the blend would be either Rose, or Helichrysum for the Leo Sun, and Pine Needle or Cypress for the Aquarius Moon. If you wanted to balance the polarities then place the blend in Number Five for Leo and Number Eleven for Aquarius, the first level of the Aura.

When you place the Oils take a moment for meditation, to infuse the action and the location with your intention and wisdom. This will raise the frequency in that part of your body and life. When we create the meditations for the Planetary Calendar, we base them on the Charts, looking for the message in each Lunation.

Of course, simply knowing the positions of the Sun and Moon is enough to create a basic meditation. For example, a good subject for the Lunation with the Leo Sun and the Aquarius Moon, would be about balancing your ego needs and your desire to participate as part of a group, to express your own genius while being open to the wisdom of others. You can use the same meditation, with the phrases reversed, at the Aquarius Sun and Leo Moon.

When you consciously interact with your surroundings, infusing it with your intentions, you make the building, the objects and the artwork instruments of your creative spirit and tools for attaining your highest purpose.

Here a couple of examples. On the New Moon in Aries place a Mars Oils in a diffuser in the Number One House representing the genetic self. Handy Mars Oils are the mints. You can make a nice blend with peppermint, pine and vanilla. This timed placement boosts personal image, self-confidence and vitality. While placing it meditate on allowing yourself to be the expressive flowering of your ancestral history.

On the New Moon in Cancer, place Cinnamon and Lemon Oil in the Number Four House, to strengthen the Hearth. At the Cancer Sun, Capricorn Moon Lunation, a nice blend is Rose Geranium and Sandalwood. Placing this in the Numbers Four and Ten Houses will help balance your desire for a well-grounded home and a satisfying career. A good meditation would be about successfully balancing your home and work life.

The Meaning of the Houses

The Sign are the actions while the Houses are where they take place, including the people and objects that are part of that experience. Each House is associated with a Sign which is listed here for reference.

The First House, Aries: The Genetics as your personal expression, core self-image, constitution and the physical body.

The Second House, Taurus: Stable personal resources, food, personal beauty and natural talents, money in the bank and real estate.

Third House, Gemini: Mobile resources, your local neighborhood, communication tools for deal making, money in the pocket, your birth language and local dialect.

Fourth House, Cancer: The hearth, kitchen, home, your matrilineal line, the places where you learn to love.

Fifth House, Leo: The places where you express yourself creatively and joyfully, places where you love romantically and playfully.

Sixth House, Virgo: Places where you work, develop skills, care for others and prepare for partnerships. Where you tend to hygiene and physical healing. The pathways and roads related to work.

Seventh House, Libra: The places and people with whom you partner and make contracts, the marriage home, shared places and where fairness is determined.

Eighth House, Scorpio: Shared resources and locations, shared power, secrets, plans, places for shared intimacy. Places for the blood mysteries and transitions.

Ninth House, Sagittarius: Places of professional training, foreign lands, places to learn foreign and professional languages, the workplaces and people who help you, and guide you towards the future, places of philosophy, enterprise and mentors.

Tenth House, Capricorn: Structures, public buildings, places connected to your career reputation, places related to people in your patrilineal line, where you achieve.

Eleventh House, Aquarius: Places where you meet others in societal networks, places for commerce, places for cooperative efforts for the common good, where you earn income from your commercial connections.

Twelfth House, Pisces: Spiritual and religious places, waterways, beaches, artist studios, where imagination rules, movie and live theaters, places of energetic healing and retreats.

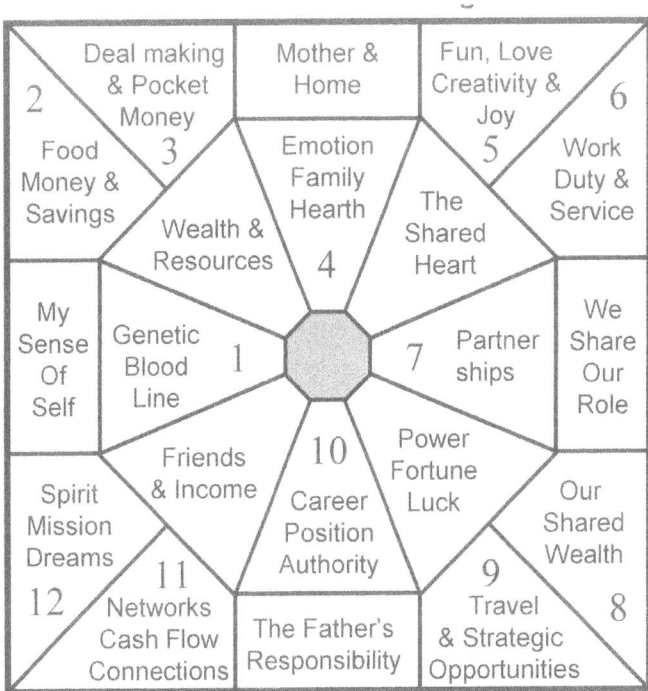

Align this Side of the Chart with the Main Door Wall

Making your enhancements with Essential Oils is like drawing a picture with a pencil, it can make a wonderful picture, but it is easy to erase. When you are ready to paint with all the colors get our books, starting with Feng Shui and the Tango in Twelve Easy Lessons and let your dreams take flight.

Note: The question of 'which is the main door' comes up so often that we have a helpful video explaining that. Visit www.spaceandtime.com/maindoor.html

The Trigrams from the I Ching or the Book of Changes

Ch'ien, Creative, Father, SUN
☰

K'un, Receptive, Mother. MOON
☷

Chen, Arousing, 1st Son, JUPITER
☳

Sun, Gentle, 1st Daughter, VENUS
☴

K'an, Abysmal, 2nd Son, SATURN
☵

Li, Clinging fire, 2nd Daughter, MARS
☲

Ken, Keeping Still, 3rd Son, EARTH
☶

Tui, Joyous, 3rd Daughter, MERCURY
☱

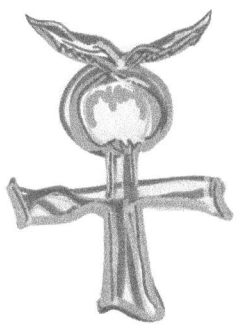

Chapter Fifteen: The Chinese Elements Explained

There should be a rule that non-astrologers cannot translate Astrological texts, because the untrained view the field simplistically and miss the complex interconnections. Project Hindsight was conceived to right this wrong with wonderful results. But, one of the places where the confusion still reigns is our western view of Chinese Astrology, whose Imperial-funded Astrological community once rivaled any in the world. When the cultural revolution obliterated that advanced scholarship, what survived, despite Mao's Little Red Book, were separate, simplified systems of Astrology, Feng Shui and Medicine.

That separation was tragic, because those three professions share philosophical foundations. When their pre-revolution texts were translated as isolated works, the translators missed the opportunity to cross check the philosophical, rather than textual meanings of the calligraphic symbols. Upon seeing a circle with five symbols; Metal, Water, Wood, Fire and Earth, they leaped to the conclusion that the system was related to the Western Astrological Elements; Fire, Earth, Air and Water. But the correlation wasn't exact.

Note: These ancient traditional Western words relate scientifically to the four states of matter; Plasma, Solid, Gaseous and Liquid. When scientific translators coopted the word 'Elements' in the 1870's, for the Russian chemist Dmitri Mendeleev's new

"Periodic Table of Elements", they borrowed legitimacy from Astrology and caused generations of confusion. It would have been more accurately translated as the Table of Periodic Atomic Weights. End of note or sidebar.

This was during a period of struggle between the Spiritualists exploring psychic events and the Scientists discovering new fundamental materials. Neither was well-informed about the other's work and they both wanted to claim the philosophical high ground. There was a one glaring problem with making that correlation of the Elements to the Chinese circle of characters, it had five symbols, not four, and it included Metal and Wood. But that was not insurmountable, because the Spiritualist philosophers were also looking at the Asian philosophies.

They justified the difference by deciding that the fifth Element related to Ether, for the spirit world. Translators expect cultural, symbolic differences and they are always happy when the numbers come out right! However, they were dramatically wrong in their assumptions! Not only did they misunderstand the significance of the characters, but then they omitted two others. It was impossible for Western Astrologers to accurately understand the Asian Astro-Medical concepts from this piecemeal system.

First, the Chinese don't call them the 'Elements', which describes a state of being. They call the characters the 'Stages', or sequential steps. That's very different! What they describe is the sequence of body systems through which a person perceives and reacts to their world, mentally, emotionally and physically.

Western Astro Medical traditions also relate body systems to the Planets, but the popular Chinese system is simpler! They start with Metal, the nervous system, leading to Water, which the emotions and autonomic reactions, then Wood, which is the structural system, then Fire, which is the muscular system and finally Earth, related to the digestive system. In the Chinese healing arts good health is seen as the unobstructed flow of activity (Chi) from one Stage to the next in this order. Disease happens when there is congestion, inflammation or depression in one of the body systems, clogging up the works and inhibiting that movement.

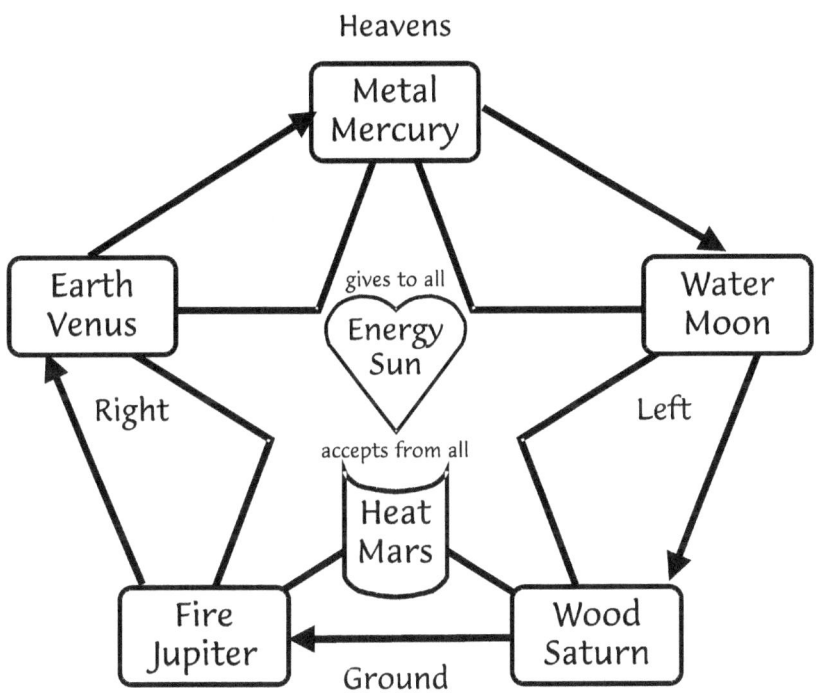

The Five Stages and Two Qualities

When a Western Medical Astrologer hears these descriptions, the correlations are obvious.

1) Metal's nervous system is Mercury.
2) Water's instinctive, emotional reaction is the Moon.
3) Wood's protective contraction is Saturn.
4) Fire's muscular expansion is Jupiter.
5) Earth's possessive processing is Venus.

This makes wonderful sense, except that the Astrology that came to us from the Greeks uses seven bodies for good reason, not five. What happened to the other two, namely the Sun and Mars? The translators left those symbols out because they were not in the circle. Fitting in two more characters was clearly a complication, when the translators were hoping for simple. They had an obvious, if imperfect correlation which made it a simple decision.

The two omitted characters are Heart Energy including circulation, which describes the Sun, and Hormonal Heat, including reproduction, which describes Mars. These two systems don't stand in line waiting to act as part of the sequence. Instead they influence and are influenced by the others. This describes how the body works; unlike the other body systems that operate on a schedule and periodically rest, the heart doesn't get any time off until the contract is up. Meanwhile, the hormonal system is reactive to changing situations, being active or dormant independent of the other system's schedules.

The Heart influences the Stages by producing high or low energy, while and Hormones affect them through producing various levels of stimulation and heat. This circle is a simple, brilliant system that describes how resources travel 'around the circle', from body system to body system. As each system becomes active it draws more Solar Energy, then when the life force moves on, its needs fall. The Chinese art of healing is about keeping the Stage's activity levels within the proper bounds. Martial Hormonal Heat is seen as problematic, because if it changes during that systems high or low ebb, it can push them out of bounds.

This ancient pattern accurately describes how the body systems interact. The Heart determines the energy level; when the heart is strong every system goes up and when it is challenged everything goes down. The heart resists challenges and multiple systems must be functioning poorly before the heart energy is depressed. In comparison, the Hormonal system doesn't have the heart's universal power, it normally affects one or two systems at a time and in turn, a problem in a single system can depress hormonal vitality.

With the Five sequential and two non-sequential body systems we see the seven traditional Planets. That is the true correlation between the Asian and Western approaches. But there's more!

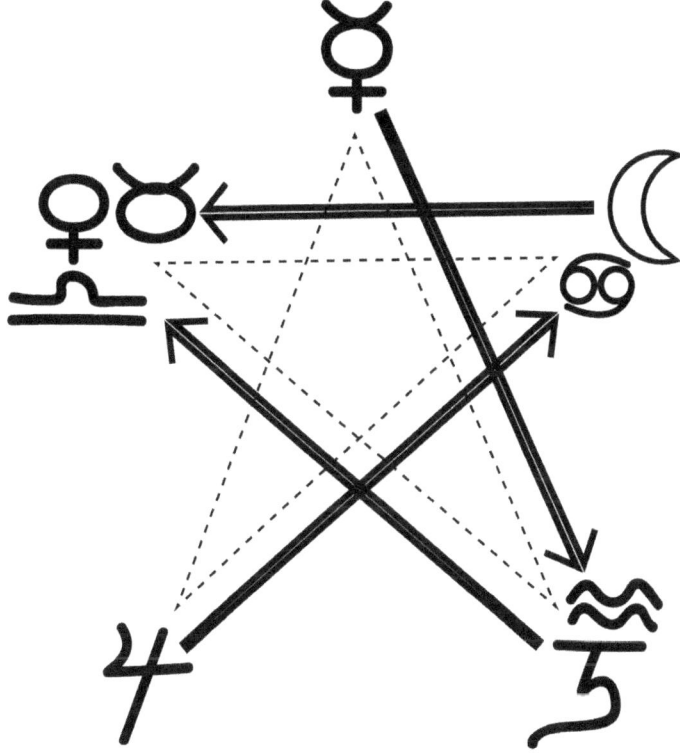

The Stages also interconnect through the alternating Planets, in a five-pointed star. Remarkably, the connections mirror some of the Exaltations from the Western Table of Dignities. The relationships are 1) Metal to Wood; which reflects Mercury's Exaltation in Saturn's traditional Dynamic Sign Aquarius. 2) Fire to Water; which reflects Jupiter's Exaltation in the Moon's Sign Cancer. 3) Wood to Earth; which reflects Saturn's Exaltation in Venus's Sign Libra. 4) Water to Earth; which reflects the Moon's Exaltation in Venus's Sign Taurus.

Planetary Exaltations describe physiological relationships. For example, the Sun is Exalted in Mars' Sign Aries, because when the heart is strong the reproductive spark is empowered. Mars is Exalted in Saturn's Sign Capricorn, because potency and fertility are dependent on a healthy mineral reserve, which is why good posture is sexually attractive.

Note: Coincidentally, the hormonal spark's best opportunities occur during Capricorn; cuddling by a wood burning fire during the long, dark nights. That's why in agricultural regions, nine months later, there are so many Virgo births. As an aside, the favorite time for country weddings is Libra, the Sign of partnerships, when the harvest bounty supports a good feast. Children conceived then are born in Gemini, Mercury's other Sign and a popular time for twin births, considered good luck for a new farming family. **End of Note**.

The differences in the two Astrological philosophies are perspective and goals. The West sees the Celestial bodies as depicting the human drama; the King, Queen and their subjects complete with their hierarchy and aspirations. The Chinese don't consider humans as central in the Universe.

When they created their systems for serving the communities, they left out something common in the West, an aspirational belief. Their society has endured for five thousand years by instructing people on how to be good members of society, but not telling them to seek advancement beyond their family's social class. It worked!

Emblematic of this is their Astrological marriage advice. Everyone in Asia knows where they fit in the twelve-year animal calendar. People are guided towards mates two or four years younger or older, so the two Jupiter positions will Sextile or Trine each other. These relationships encourage a financially stable family.

They are warned against a three-year difference, the Jupiter Square, because it would challenge them to achieve more, with an accompanying risk of loss. The ideal Chinese coupling results in stability! Admittedly, in five thousand years they noticed some finer points and there are preferred pairings. For example, two Rabbits are supposed to make a good match, probably because of the bunny's prolific tendencies.

The Chinese practically invented the concept of proprietary products; their systems are often so opaque to outsiders that it's amazing that the early translators accomplished as much as they did. Our 'Rosetta Stone' was the comparison of the Asian and Western Astrological views of human physiology. Astrology is ultimately a practical approach to nature, and we have found that human bodies, no matter what part of the globe they walk on, share the same divine design.

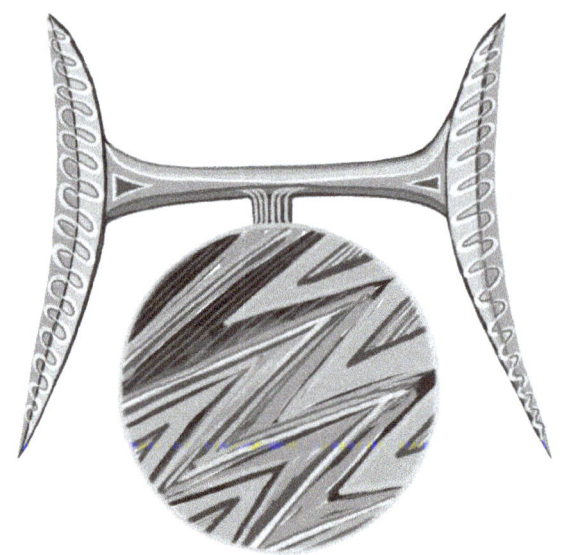

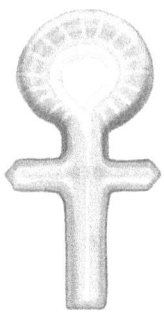

Chapter Sixteen: The Visible Planets and the Invisible You

Astrologer- Ah, you're one of those people! Client- What people? Astrologer- You're one of those people who navigate by the Stars that others don't see!

Why are some people's talents recognized early, while others struggle to gather support for their interests? That difference is determined by which category of Planets are in the first five Houses of the Chart. Why? Because that sequence of the early Houses describes the steps in which we encounter the world. The first three Houses, like the first three years of life, are instinctive, autonomic and practically undeniable, while in the fourth and fifth Houses those instill responses that move beyond the instinctual physical to the emotional.

Here are the steps through which we encounter the world: We meet others with our Ascendant in the Martial First House; determining if they are a man, woman, child, big, little or equal in size? The important measurement we use is the level of threat they represent! In the Venusian Second House we note their strength, beauty, clothing and scent. In the Mercurial Third House, we identify how they communicate, their touch, accent, body language and style. In the Lunar Fourth House we go beyond our tactile experience to find out about their family and where they live. In the Solar Fifth House we sense their heart.

What are these categories of Planets? There are two! The first group has been known to humanity for eons because they can be seen with the naked eye. The Sun, Moon, Mercury, Venus, Mars, Jupiter and Saturn are the 'Visible Planets'. The second category are those Planets that are only seen with the help of a telescope; Uranus, Neptune and Pluto. Most people have never personally 'seen' them and are only aware of them through photos. We call this group the 'Invisible Planets' and it includes, to a lesser importance, the major Asteroids.

There is a fundamental difference between how humans experience these two groups; the 'Visibles' are right there in the sky, with nothing in between. Watching Venus before dawn rising in the East is a memorable experience, felt in your gut and your soul. The 'Invisibles' are hidden in the blackness of night and even through a telescope, it's hard to make that soulful connection.

Don't underestimate the power of personal perception. Imagine the experiential difference between watching a news story on the television, compared to running for your car, carrying a hastily packed bag, because the forest fire that you smelled before you saw the glow, is now coming down the hill. Dramatically different!

Part of that disconnect also comes from the long timelines of the Invisibles. We connect emotionally and physically with the Moon because the quickly changing Phases affect us on numerous levels, including most notably the tides and the amount of Moon light we enjoy. The Visible Planet with the longest timeline, Saturn, has a twenty-eight-year orbit, an age that most people, even in ancient cultures, expected to reach.

In comparison, the 84 years it takes Uranus to orbit the Sun is twelve years longer than the average person's life span. If that's hard to grasp, the 165-years for Neptune to make the circuit of the twelve Signs, and 248-years for Pluto's voyage are like mythical ideas to most people. The last time that Pluto was in the current Sign people were traveling in horse drawn carriages and depending on oil lamps!

The category of Planets leading in those early Houses indicate whether or not a person will likely receive early validation for their interests. If it is filled with 'Visible Planets', others recognize that child's interests early and the child reacts enthusiastically to that support.

When those early Houses are led by the 'Invisible Planets', the person's interests are more difficult for others to recognize, like very dim points in a dark night sky. Unless their elders possess that 'difficult to see' interest themselves, the esoteric equivalent of a telescope, that child's true interests may go unnoticed. Fortunately, talents, along with debilities can be hereditary, so sometimes a family member may recognize that unique interest, like the psychic Aunt who senses their niece's special gift, to which the parents are mostly oblivious.

When the person has the 'Visibles' (the Sun, Moon and Planets out to Saturn) leading the charge they are initially drawn to obvious (aka visible) interests that society supports, so support is readily available.

For example, a child with Mars in the First House is drawn to physical activity and will happily walk into new situations and meet new people. Those around him will value that talent and let them be the lead in those kinds of situations. Because they receive validation for those actions, and get the opportunity to develop those skills, they enjoy filling that role that other people readily recognize and appreciate.

When the person has the 'Invisibles' leading the charge, they are attracted to interests beyond the common perception of most people, so family and teachers are not quick to validate their primary interests. For example, if a child has Invisible Neptune in the First House, their gifts for imagination and visualization are awesome, but internalized, so others don't recognize them. They may see that child as a daydreamer, but what that child is looking for is the unifying story in what they see. However, in this world where visible accomplishments are the rule, that gift requires a special condition in order to be acknowledged. Often the leading Invisible Planet is passed over in favor of the next 'Visible Planet' in the lineup.

This is like picking teams in grammar school, where the team captains pick their friends first, passing over the kids whose skills they don't know. If that Invisible Neptune in the first House is followed by a strong Visible Venus in the Second House, the child's natural beauty, charm and artistic talent will be encouraged, even while their boundless imagination is ignored.

That doesn't mean that those Venusian gifts are not one of the child's interests, a well-placed Venus is an undeniable force, but that is not what they wake up in the morning thinking about, Neptune is!

Because Venus is not primary interest, the adults will be surprised by the child's lack of automatic enthusiasm for their support. But children respond to encouragement and they'll eventually summon what the elders considers a sufficient response.

The challenge is that a Planetary talent can be expressed in multiple arenas, with that Venus in the Second House they could be guided towards the arts, but also to working in restaurants, banking, real estate or agriculture; professions where the Neptune would feel stifled.

When a child is offered support that takes all those qualities into account they will bloom, and their enthusiasm will soar. The strategy will hopefully avoid the odd journey where someone completes an education in one field, only to pursues a career in a completely different area in alignment with their true interests.

Here is an example on the opposite page of the conventional acceptance that comes from having the 'visible' Planets leading. Super salesman and Presidential candidate **Ross Perot,** like many successful salespeople, was born near dawn, with important players at the Ascendant.

It wired him to bring BIG energy to his initial contacts with people, a quality recognized early, even though he stood only 5'5" tall! Having Pluto embedded with the bigger players supercharged the mix and added the global view that you would think a Presidential candidate ought to have, coming from Pluto's long orbit.

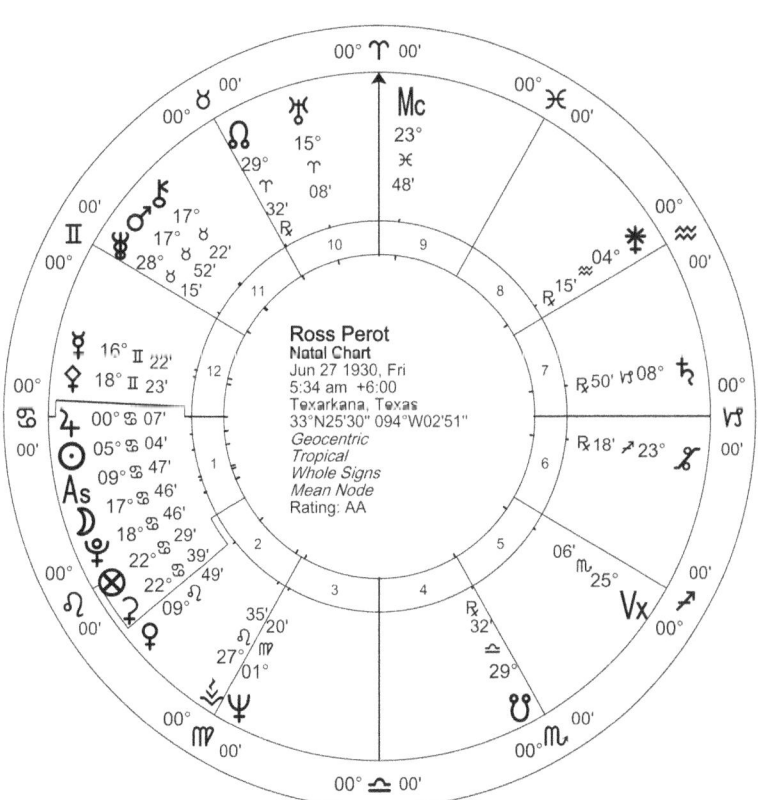

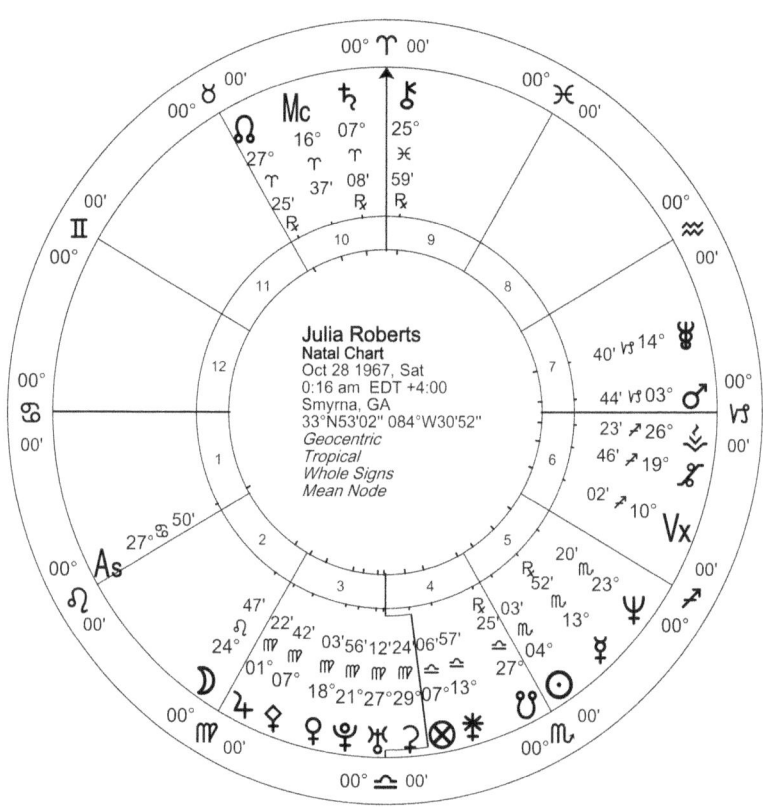

But the emphasis does not have to be near the Ascendant to garner acceptance. The actress **Julia Roberts** makes an immediate impression from the Second House. Her Moon at 24 degrees Leo commands the Cancer Ascendant, projecting a glowing femininity and a sense of innate talent.

This is supported by a Visible Jupiter at the Royal Star Regulus, and a very feminine Virgo Venus in the Third. She was sensitized by these three visible leading Planets, which led to her first blockbuster role at age 23, 'Pretty Woman'.

Uranus, Neptune and Pluto in those leading spots act very differently. A solitary leading Neptune impels the person to seek the spiritual story in every situation, but that Neptunian 'vision' is often missed by others. A sole leading Uranus instills an alternate viewpoint, thanks to its odd spin, that is easy to miss.

The solitary Pluto gives an interest in global events and long timelines, but requires a long maturation period, often causing career delays or detours, as seen in the following example.

Pope Francis has Pluto in Cancer Rising giving him a global view, with Neptune in Virgo in the Third House, making him want to share his Spiritual narrative. But, as a child people noticed his first visible Planet, a Fourth House Mars in Libra, the aggressive peacekeeper.

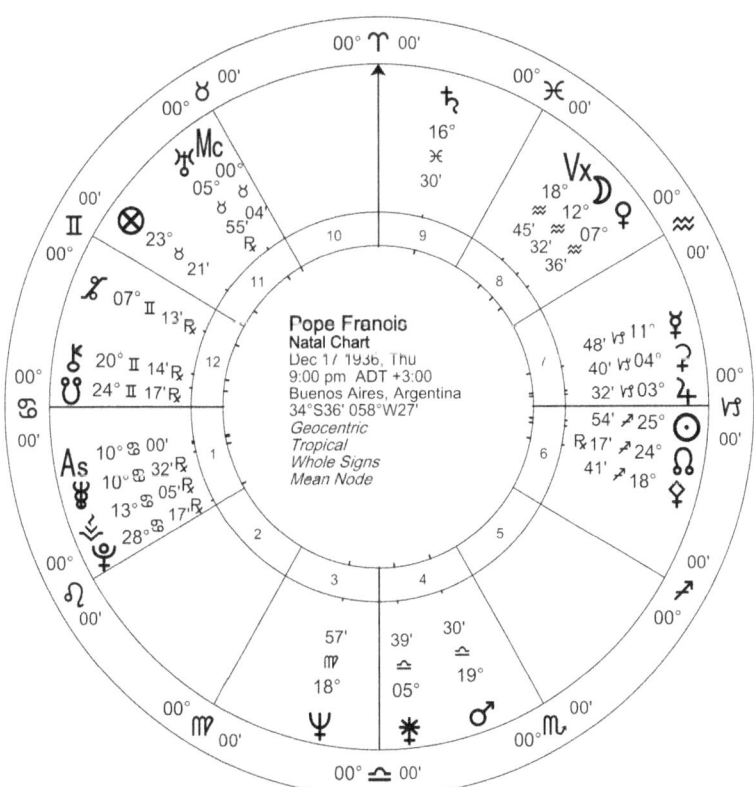

That's the kid who fearlessly stands between fighting classmates on the playground; his peacemaker skills are still evident today. His visible, philosophical Sun in Sagittarius, in the Sixth House, at the esoteric Galactic Center, with the visible Eighth House Aquarius Moon, commanding his Ascendant from the managerial Eighth House, gives him the clear mark of the shepherd.

Due to those visible Planets he was guided to a pastoral career with a congregation, instead of as an administrator; the path preferred by the ambitious churchmen. Even though they were hidden, those leading invisible Planets gave Francis the dedication and visionary flair to be a global leader. Because a Pope ascends the throne late in life, for Francis at age 76, he had time to manifest those far-reaching 'invisible' energies.

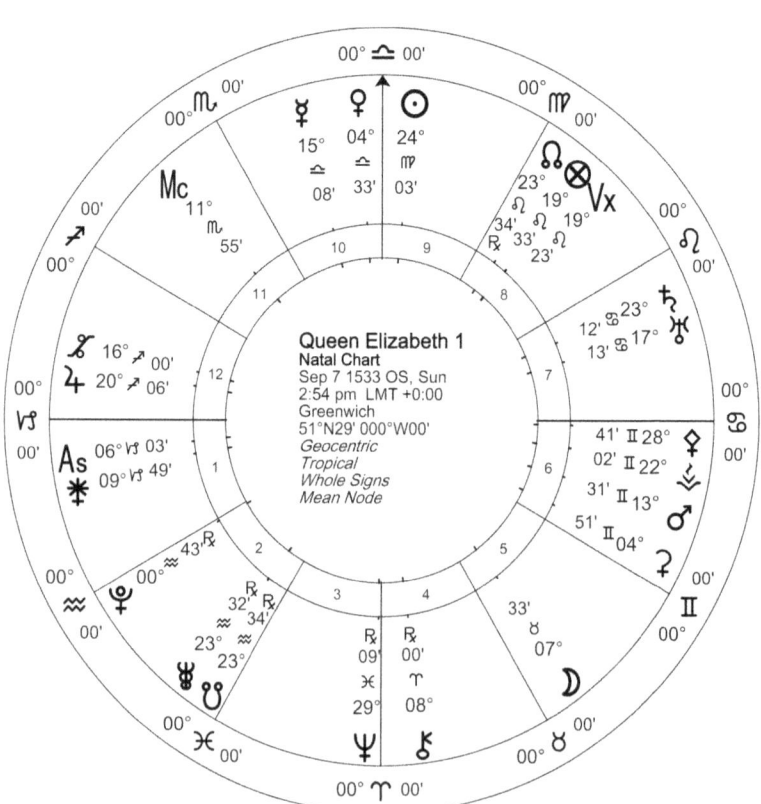

The 'Virgin Queen' **Elizabeth the First**, had a similar line up. While she ascended the throne early, political and religious challengers made her appear a very temporary resident of the English throne. But once she had leverage, the strategic global view provided by her Second House Pluto, with her Third House Neptune's deep belief. That was coupled with a Twelfth House, entrepreneurial Jupiter in Sagittarius. That inspired her funding of Neptune's Navy, her adventurous sea Captains, that helped turn her forty-four-year reign into a golden age.

The Invisibles don't need to cling to the Ascendant to create this effect, it is the House sequence that matters. If the first two Houses are empty, but a leading Uranus is in the Third, that might produce dyslexia, or the ability to see auras, which other people might never know about. Conservative societies fearfully suppress the messages of those Planets beyond the Saturnian wall, because they represent forces outside of their control.

That's why artists and actors move to big cities, or people with niche interests visit chat groups; they are seeking opportunities to express the interests that their local circle fails to recognize. The challenge is partially ameliorated when the leading Invisible Planet is paired with a Visible body, that acts as a patron for its mysterious friend, opening doors of acceptance.

This is like having a good friend visit your home, who brings along their cousin, visiting from another country. You've never met this stranger before, with their exotic accent and interesting clothes, but because they are part of your friend's family, you welcome them. They in turn introduce you to a unique perspective of the world.

The most problematic situations are when the Invisibles dominate the personal Houses from one to six, while the Visible bodies fill the social Houses, seven to twelve. The person's public life can't help but steal their personal thunder, making it difficult to pursue their primary interests. The first six Houses is where the person's unique character traits and responses develop. Because their inner experience is invisible to those around them, and thus not actively engaged by others, it may stunt their emotional and spiritual growth. It may require a life-changing event to empower them, or force them, to explore that inner life.

This can describe those popular, social young people who suddenly self-destruct. Like all of us, they needed to share their essential perceptions and attractions, but that need was overshadowed by their activities in 'the visible world', so no one was listening. This makes the case for young people spending significant time traveling outside of their constrictive social circle, to help them find a voice for their primary interests.

Noting whether the leading Planets in a Chart are Visible or Invisible, to determine how people are seen by the world is simple to do. You can offer those who navigate by the Stars that others don't see, validation for pursuing their uniquely satisfying life interests, despite the lack of previous external guidance. Astrologers can provide this valuable perspective for the simple reason that we have telescopes, and we know how to use them.

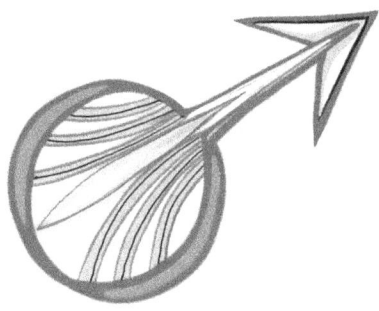

Chapter Seventeen: The Astrology of Fine Wine

"Wine is sunlight held together by water" - Galileo Galilei

In 1811 the "Great Comet" was visible for over eight months, and the year's wine was called a "Comet Vintage". That year's flawless Château d'Yquem enjoyed exceptional longevity, the Veuve Clicquot was heralded as the first 'modern' Champagne and while 1811 stands out, all of the 'comet vintages' are believed exceptional.

Our consulting spans both Astrology and wine tourism, places where the history of natural cycles rule, so we divide our time talking with clients about their Planets and the vineyards that produce the wines they like. A person's wine preferences are often expressions of their Charts, accounting for differences in age, economic status, education, gender and physiology. Personal transits affect what appeals to their palates and the travel experiences people seek. Saturn Transits often inspire wine trips to Bordeaux, with all their formality and tradition. Jupiter Transits more often lead to bouncing among the California vineyards, with the hospitable, over-blown and entrepreneurial style.

Three factors shape wine preferences; personality, physiology and age. Astrologically, Personality is the Sun and Moon, Physiology is the Ascendant and Age is seen in the transits. Older men and Saturnian personalities like big, structured, aged Reds. Youngsters, before their Saturn Return at the age of twenty-eight, often like lighter, even sweeter wines that delight and excite the front of the palette. As people age the flavors that appeal to them are sensed farther back on the palate. After the Saturn Return, the mid-palette, savory flavors of calcium, magnesium, sodium and potassium become more appealing. At that critical juncture the body's ability to assimilate these nutrients is reduced, so it becomes increasingly important that the body seek them out.

Herbalists have traditionally made correlations between plants and Planets. With grapes that's easy, because they look like Celestial Bodies, round, colorful with distinctive personalities. Having our unique perspective, we looked for correlations between the major Planets and the grapes that dominate the 'fine wine' world.

Here is a helpful hint for wine lovers from Biodynamics, the oldest, 'modern' system of organic farming, that includes an Astrological system. Wine is more fragrant and tastes better during Fire and Air Moons, compared to Water and Earth Moons. That's because the flavors volatize more easily under those Moons.

A major part of the sensory enjoyment of wine is through the nose, which can detect almost a billion scent notes, while the palate only gets five major flavors. We have noticed this ourselves and the Moon Sign is an important factor for when the great Biodynamic French wine houses schedule their industry tasting events.

The Celestial Bodies and Their Grapes

The Sun – Chardonnay. When that golden glass of Chardonnay is glowing in the café light you are seeing the embodiment of the Sun. The name in Persian means 'The Gates of Heaven', and as befits the Sun, Chard is America's biggest selling premium white wine; climate tolerant, insect resistant, prolific and able to be made in many styles. Like all grapes, they start off green but as they attain ripeness, they become a translucent gold, with subtle sunspots floating beneath the surface. That vitality and adaptability is clearly Solar.

The Moon – Moscato. This grape is a large golden globe, a touch speckled and sometimes colored a soft rose all over; fragrant, watery and inclined to a high sugar level. How feminine and Lunar is that? Doubling as a table grape, it's a special seasonal treat.

Inside the winery Moscato flashes multiple faces, from its famous sweet wine, to a bright, dry glass that still retains its trace of perfume. It likes to be part of a family and is often mixed with other wines to add some 'nose' and softness, especially with stiff Chardonnay and the Mercurial Pinot Blanc, to create what the French call their White Burgundy.

Mercury - Pinot Noir and Pinot Blanc are the two faces of Mercury, small, delicate grapes growing beside Solar Chardonnay. The name 'Pinot', for the 'Pine' cone shaped bunches, the source of pine nuts, makes sense because these grapes drive growers nuts, with their challenges; something they have in common with Mercury ruled people.

Pinot Blanc is rarely made as a single wine. A bit thin in personality, it has the wonderful ability to reflect and complement another grape's gifts with those famous Gemini engaging skills. Even Pinot Noir, which is made as a single grape, is often a mix of various 'clones' or mutations from varied vineyards, like a troupe of Virgos, working together to accomplish a task.

As easy as Chard is to grow, the Pinot twins are more troublesome, thin-skinned, sensitive to everything and even at their best, their yields, like their berries and the Planet Mercury, are small. **Venus – Riesling.** Few wines bring a smile to the lips as quickly as Riesling because of its light body, bright fragrance and sweet flavor, it often appeals to younger palates. For many people this grape from the northlands is the first glass that opened their eyes to the possibilities of wine. How much like Venus is that, the power of love, beauty and attraction to make you notice something that you had, up until then, overlooked.

Growing Riesling is a labor of love because it thrives in very specific locations where other grapes would not. Like all grapes, it needs plenty of sunlight, but its thin, light-colored skin lets it ripen quicker than most. To grow a good Riesling in these cooler climates, they pick the warmest spots with the most sunshine; steep, terraced, southern facing hillside vineyards overlooking the river. The amount of effort and care required for those remarkable locations seems out of proportion to their results, but that's what people will do for the sake of Venus.

Mars – Malbec. The connection between Mars and hormones is clear, because both are powerful, sociable, sure to get your attention, but short lived. Interestingly, according to Biodynamics Mars is considered the most important Planet for growing grapes because of their similar ruddy complexions, as most grapes are red. Malbec possesses a rich flavor, great color, but low tannins, which makes it a favorite with women, fitting perfectly with Mars Ruled Scorpio, the Sign of strong women.

Even though Mars is Earth's neighbor, it is half the size of Venus and twice as far from Earth. That is like Malbec, which historically comes from the small Cohors Valley, to the east of the much larger, richer Bordeaux region. But small is still potent and the 'Black Wine of Cohors' was especially prized by the ancient Romans and Czarist Russia, two Martial societies.

Jupiter – Merlot. The big, juicy Merlot berry makes a richly flavored, well-rounded wine with fruity flavors, but very low amounts of the tannins that pucker your lips. This sounds so much like how we describe the abundantly appealing nature of huge Jupiter. Merlot became an early favorite when single varietal wines became popular because the flavors opened and became accessible quickly and it went well with so many foods.

Like Jupiter's two Signs, Sagittarius and Pisces, Merlot is a very social wine and an early favorite in the bar scene. That's because 'Merlot' was easier to pronounce in front of a young lady than Cabernet Sauvignon, Sangiovese or Gewürztraminer.

Merlot's burgeoning popularity produced too much mediocre wine, until the movie 'Sideways', where the main character rails against the grape, dramatically damaging sales. That was like the comet Hale Bopp slamming into Jupiter! But Merlot, like Jove, is hard to keep down and Merlot's quality and popularity, thanks to better vineyard strategies, has gradually rebounded.

Saturn – Cabernet Sauvignon. Saturn is the old man of the ancient Planets, taking twenty-eight years to orbit the Sun and Cabernet is one of the last vines to flower, the last to harvest and the more time it has on the vines and in the bottle the better it tastes. Cab loves the sun, dry weather and well-drained soils, high in sulfur, to make tannins that give Cabernet its ability to survive in the cellars.

That Saturnian durability is why it commands high prices. It is the banker's wine because you put it in your cellar and it increases in value, year after year. Buy a Cabernet the year a child is born and enjoy it with them on their twenty-first birthday, or better yet, at their Saturn Return.

Cabernets, like Saturn with its spectacular rings, is renowned for its beauty, sporting deeply colored reds with a flickering of other hues as the glass's level descends. While young people find those tannins and complex flavors overwhelming, older men, with less sensitive, but more experienced palettes, appreciate the strongly structured flavors that their bodies crave.

Uranus – Viognier. Both the Planet and the Wine make deceptive first impressions. Uranus was long mistaken for a Star until the 1700's when it was revealed as a Planet. But then, Surprise! Its odd nature was revealed. Unlike the other Planets that stand upright, spinning like a top, Uranus rotates on its East-West axis, sailing through space like a well thrown football.

Viognier also surprises because its floral scent doesn't foretell the structured, full-bodied wine on your palette. Uranus is the only planet beyond Saturn, that given ideal conditions, can be seen without a telescope. Viognier had almost died out but was rescued from obscurity by the Central Coast winemakers seeking "ABC wines", for people who want "Anything But Chardonnay", that would thrive in their cool, windy hills. Uranus is also considered the Alternative Planet. Those winemakers were so tired of making tank after tank of Chardonnay that the alternative, Viognier, even though difficult and demanding to make, was a welcome change.

Neptune – Zinfandel. The Planet and the Wine are both mysterious, often defying description and are favorites in California. With the state's long Pacific coastline and spectacular harbors, Neptune, the God of the Seas, clearly holds sway. Zinfandel was long thought a 'native' Californian grape, an emotion that persists despite genetic testing claims from coastal Croatia, but with Neptune, feelings matter more than facts! Neptune's influence is nebulous, acting behind the scenes, it is associated with the imagination, alcohol and drugs, and it is an important 'money' Planet.

That's like Zinfandel, it has an unusual combination of qualities; both full body and deep color, but the grapes are early ripening, so it comes to the market early. That's why Zin was so popular during Prohibition, when tons of grapes were shipped to the big East Coast cities, the earlier your grapes made it to the train yards, the better chance you had of selling every bunch. Zin is often made in a very intoxicating, high alcohol version.

Like Neptune, Zin often lives in the background, a durable vine, whose deep roots are hidden from view. Its grapes are often included, but unacknowledged, in inexpensive red blends. Neptune also travels beyond the reach of the naked eye, ruling those who make movies, video games and wine, so just like Zinfandel, Neptune is perfectly at home in the Virgo Ruled Golden State.

Pluto - Petite Verdot. This is the small, dark grape, whose name means 'The little green one'. It is mostly added to red Bordeaux blends to replace tannins and colors washed out of the Cabernet grapes by early rains. Without those components the wine won't age properly. It is rarely made by itself, but fermented alone it is a profoundly dark, appealing red wine. That is so like Pluto, a Planet smaller than Earth's Moon, but with five Moons of its own, invisible to the naked eye, traveling on its long Solar orbit through the depths of space.

It adds depth and intensity to the chart through its Conjunctions with other Planets. Petite Verdot also has a long timeline, ripening late in the season, and making its invisible presence known by helping the wines extend their lives years into the future. Pluto, thanks to its long orbit, is also about the historical perspective. It teaches us about the purposes and limitations of power, a lesson that is most often learned later in life.

Wine is one of the proofs that God
loves us and wants us to be happy
- Benjamin Franklin, Astrologer and Statesman
Well said Ben!

166 Planetary Calendar Astrology

The Planetary Calendar

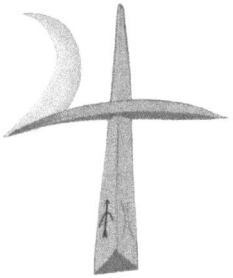

Watch
Forecasting Videos & Educational @ www.SpaceAndTime.com

The Brief Monthly Videos Expand
on the Planetary Calendar Forecasts.

Learn to use the Calendar's Data and Information
in your Daily Life with the 'How To' Videos, and
The Astro Minutes. These average about 10 Minutes
and address various practical and technical subjects.

Including:

A Walk Around the Signs, the 12 Seasons
Understanding Planetary Glyphs and what they symbolize
Get to Know the Big Three Markers, Sun, Moon & Rising
Recognizing the Moon's Motions, the fastest player
Using Planetary Rulerships, who has the upper hand?
Calculating Aspects, how the planets interact
Looking at Retrograde Planets, when they appear to back up
Visualize the Fixed Stars, the 'unchanging' sky
How the Chinese Signs relate to the Western Signs
Calendars, do we understand them?

Watch Episodes of Planetary Calendar Astrology & Astrologers Chatting Over Coffee @ www.PlanetaryCalendar.com

First Episode: The show's New Format
Second Episode: The Calendar's New Healing Features
Third Episod: The Chart of Starbucks and its Founder
Fourth Episode: The Connections Between Wine and the Stars
Fifth Episode: The Astrology of the Movie Justice League
Sixth Episode: The Democratic Presidential Candidates
Seventh Episode: TV's Most Popular Drama, Why it Works!

You Can Also Find Videos Related to Herbal Healing and Essential Oils in The 10 Minute Herbalist Section

You Can Find Videos Related to Feng Shui and Geomancy in the Ask Ralph & Lahni Section

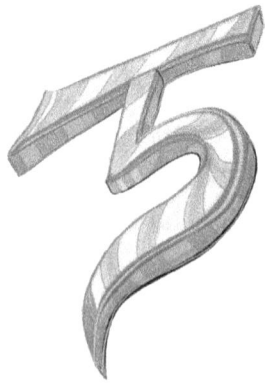

Book & Calendar Catalog & Orders

Feng Shui and the Tango, The Dance of Design
Do you want more fun, romance, commitment, acclaim and improved cash flow? The book shows you how to program your surroundings for attaining what you want. 288 pages, $17.99. The 'Tango' Series includes Prosperity Lessons & Happiness Lessons.

The Dream Desk Quiz, Improving Personal & Team Performance Through Recognizing Your Ergo Dynamic Personality. Seven multiple choice questions and forty-three personalized answers to help unleash your talents, leadership skills and team cooperation. 92 pages, $9.95.

Creating Clarity, The Incredibly Simple, Surprisingly Surefire Solution to Clutter! It is easier than you think. The key is understanding the underlying ergonomic causes and then changing them! 92 pages, $9.95

The 10 Minute Herbalist, This collection of short chapters gets right to the point with solutions that help resolve many of today's most persistent health problems, based on forty years plus of practical experience. 148 pages, $12.95

A Year of Healthful Hints, Ideas for Living a Healthy Life. Started as a weekly email, this has a feminine approach; caring, entertaining and insightful. The 70 chapters are easy to understand, effective natural solutions for today's health problems. 192 pages $12.95

Good Health is Easy, It's Being Sick That's Rough! Eight chapters that are the foundation of Ralph & Lahni's Aloe to Zingiber Master Herbalist program, with essential information for maintaining good health using Natural methods. 222 pages $12.95

Planetary Calendar Astrology, Moving Beyond Observation Into Action. Designed as a companion to the Calendar, it includes an entertaining introduction to Astrological principles and various powerful Location and Healing techniques that the authors use in their practice and forecasts. $19.95.

Order Books & Calendars at www.SpaceAndTime.com

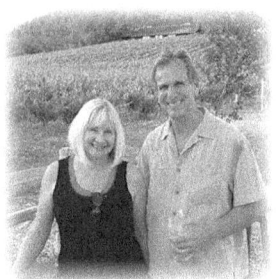

About the Authors
Ralph & Lahni DeAmicis

Ralph & Lahni had both maintained low profiles as professional astrologers, working independently since the early 1970s, not having met each other until 1994. When they first showed up as speakers on the International Astrological scene in the mid-1990s, with their insightful, entertaining, 'tag-team' presentations, people asked, "Where did you guys come from?"

That meeting in 1994 was in the Physics Lab at the pivotal Project Hindsight Conference, at Princeton University. The stars aligned and they fell in love and formed a consulting practice called Space and Time Designing, to address their client's astrological and environmental design issues, which at that point were becoming increasingly popular due to the arrival of Feng Shui in the West.

Very quickly, they became popular speakers at International Feng Shui and Astrological conferences, while their consulting practice grew. Then they began writing books together! Their first book was called "From Gaia with Love, A Guide to Astro Herbology". This was inspired by their interest in the spiritual side of natural healing.

Their second book was called, "Feng Shui and the Tango in 12 Easy Lessons", now in its fourth edition. This book was unique in that genre because it integrated Classic Asian Feng Shui with Western Astrology and Geomancy. Next, they wrote "The 10 Minute Herbalist", a collection of short chapters addressing many of today's health challenges.

Both 'Tango' and "The 10 Minute Herbalist" kicked off two series of books on those topics. But, until now, Ralph and Lahni had not written any other Astrology books, despite becoming well known for their work in Locational and Health Astrology. They had written articles and monthly magazine forecasts and their Annual Global Chinese New Year Forecast has become a perennial favorite. Then clients and students begged for them to write books.

In 1998, after the passing of the originator, they became the second astrologers of the "Planetary Calendar", which had been published continuously since 1949. That mostly required making the calculations, summations and judgements for each day and putting them in a standardized format. But, with a little encouragement, the publisher agreed to let them include a monthly forecast which gradually led to other minor improvements.

In 2012 Ralph and Lahni began producing a monthly TV show called Planetary Calendar, based on those forecasts, featuring Lahni and the then publisher, her daughter, Carole Cherry. Over time, Ralph took over as the second astrologer, recreating the 'Ralph & Lahni show" from their speaking days. In 2020 it was rebranded 'Astrologers Chatting Over Wine'. The show's format included a second segment on educational astrology topics. Eventually the format evolved into full episodes dedicated to topical subjects: business, entertainment, politics, chart analysis and more. The expanded monthly forecasts are available on the website, **www.SpaceAndTime.com**. In 2018 Ralph and Lahni took over as the publishers of Planetary Calendar, using their design skills to make numerous improvements in this long running almanac. They realized that there were additional astrological concepts that they wanted the calendar's devoted readers to understand, which led to their writing their first book on this subject in over 20 years, "Planetary Calendar Astrology".

You can contact them through the www.SpaceAndTime.com website

Ordering Books & Next Year's Planetary Calendars & Day Planners

Calendars are ready in the Summer of the current year. Advance orders are mailed as soon as the calendars are available. They can be purchased on the website, or prepaid with a check, money order or credit card. Please include your contact info in case there are questions about your order. Consult the website for the complete catalog and new products.

Order Online at www.PlanetaryCalendar.com

In the USA: **Large Wall Size** 8.5" x 11" $20.00, **Medium Wall Size** 7" x 9" $18.00, **Pocket Size** 4.5" x 5.5" $15.00, **Day Planner** 5.5" x 8.5", 218 pgs $22.00
Planetary Calendar Astrology 5.5" x 8.5", 172 pgs $20.00

Canada & Mexico: **Large Wall Size** 8.5" x 11" $20.00, **Medium Wall Size** 7" x 9" $20.00, **Pocket Size** 4.5" x 5.5" $7.00, **Day Planner** 5.5" x 8.5", 218 pages $25.00
Planetary Calendar Astrology 5.5" x 8.5", 172 pgs $23.00

Mail Orders to:
Planetary Calendar
PO Box 5391
Napa, CA 94581-0391

For Phone Orders or Customer Service leave a Voicemail at **(800) 217-4197**. We accept AmEx, Disc, MC or Visa via Phone & Online. Credit card orders require full name, billing address, phone number & email along with credit card #, exp date, & security code. Shipping and Handling is included.

Please allow 4-6 weeks for delivery, although they are typically shipped immediately. Not responsible for postal delays.

Planetary Calendar Published Since 1949

roduct-compliance